ACPL, Laramie, WY   08/2017
000400765096
The Battle against infection /
Pieces: 1

D0461440

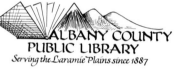

ALBANY COUNTY
PUBLIC LIBRARY
Serving the Laramie Plains since 1887

Laramie, Wyoming 82070

PRESENTED BY

A Friend

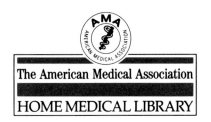

The American Medical Association

HOME MEDICAL LIBRARY

THE BATTLE
AGAINST
INFECTION

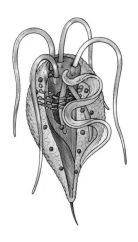

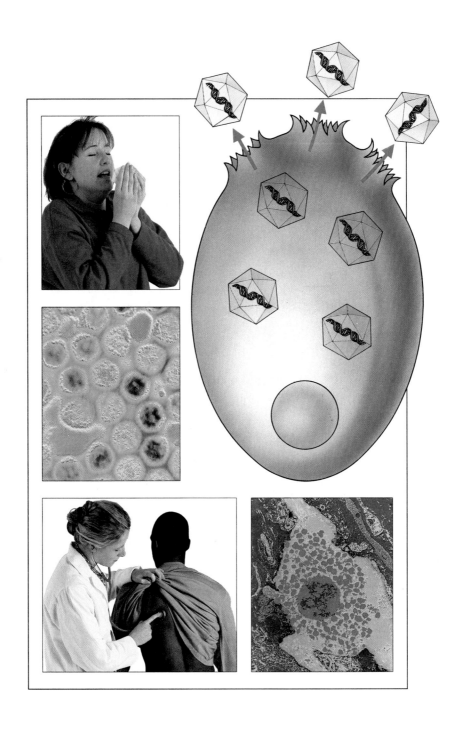

THE AMERICAN
MEDICAL ASSOCIATION

THE BATTLE
AGAINST
INFECTION

Medical Editor
CHARLES B. CLAYMAN, MD

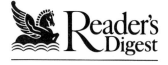
Reader's Digest

THE READER'S DIGEST ASSOCIATION, INC.
Pleasantville, New York/Montreal

WITHDRAWN

ALBANY COUNTY
PUBLIC LIBRARY
LARAMIE, WYOMING

The AMA Home Medical Library was created and produced
by Dorling Kindersley, Ltd., in association with the
American Medical Association.

Copyright © 1992 Dorling Kindersley, Ltd., and
American Medical Association

Copyright © 1992 Text Dorling Kindersley, Ltd., and
American Medical Association

Copyright © 1992 Illustrations Dorling Kindersley, Ltd.

All rights reserved under International and
Pan-American Copyright Conventions. Published in the
United States by The Reader's Digest Association, Inc.,
Pleasantville, New York/Montreal

Manufactured in the United States of America

The information in this book reflects current medical knowledge. The
recommendations and information are appropriate in most cases;
however, they are not a substitute for medical diagnosis. For specific
information concerning your personal medical condition, the AMA
suggests that you consult a physician.

The names of organizations, products, or alternative therapies appearing
in this book are given for informational purposes only. Their inclusion
does not imply AMA endorsement, nor does the omission of any
organization, product, or alternative therapy indicate AMA disapproval.

The AMA Home Medical Library is distinct from and unrelated to the
series of health books published by Random House, Inc., in conjunction
with the American Medical Association under the names "The AMA Home
Reference Library" and "The AMA Home Health Library."

Library of Congress Cataloging in Publication Data

The Battle against infection / medical editor, Charles B. Clayman.
     p. cm — (The American Medical Association home
medical library)
    At head of title: The American Medical Association.
    Includes index.
    ISBN 0-89577-412-7
    1. Communicable diseases — Popular works. 2. Infection — Popular
works.   I. Clayman, Charles B. II. American Medical Association.
III. Series.
  [DNLM: 1. Infection — prevention & control — popular works.
2. Microbiology — popular works. WC 195 B336]
RC113.B28 1992
616.9 — dc20
DNLM/DLC
for Library of Congress   91-42001

READER'S DIGEST and the Pegasus logo are registered trademarks of
The Reader's Digest Association, Inc.

FOREWORD

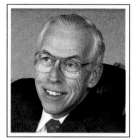

As recently as the first half of this century, many young adults died of diseases such as tuberculosis, polio, and diphtheria. At the same time, almost every child acquired common childhood infections, including measles, mumps, and whooping cough. Most children survived these illnesses, but many did not. Today the situation is much improved, thanks to advances in nutrition and living standards and the development of lifesaving vaccines and antibiotics. With the exception of AIDS, which confounds doctors and researchers alike, infectious diseases are no longer life-threatening to most Americans. Nevertheless, infections still cause illness for many people. Children get frequent colds, sore throats, and ear infections. There have been recent outbreaks of measles because many children have not been immunized, underscoring the need for vaccinations. Most adults have at least one respiratory or digestive tract infection each year. The incidence of sexually transmitted diseases continues to climb at an astounding rate.

Early recognition of the cause of an infection and prompt and appropriate treatment usually shorten the length of illness and reduce the risk of complications. This volume of the AMA Home Medical Library gives you practical advice on how you can minimize your risk of infection. When you do get sick, this book will help you determine if you need to see your doctor or if you can treat your illness at home.

Although many infections still cannot be cured, doctors today have a much better understanding of what causes them and how they affect us. Once a disease organism has been identified, scientists can develop effective vaccines or drugs to prevent or treat the specific infection that it causes. New techniques in genetic engineering are making it easier to produce safe and effective synthetic vaccines against serious infections such as viral hepatitis. We can say with confidence that science is winning the battle against infection.

JAMES S. TODD, MD
Executive Vice President
American Medical Association

THE AMERICAN
MEDICAL ASSOCIATION

James S. Todd, MD — *Executive Vice President*
Wendy Borow — *Vice President, Consumer Publishing*
Heidi Hough — *Publisher, Consumer Books*

EDITORIAL STAFF

Charles B. Clayman, MD — *Medical Editor*
Dorothea Guthrie — *Managing Editor*
Lori A. Barba — *Senior Editor*
Pam Brick — *Senior Editor*
Donna Kotulak — *Senior Editor*
Patricia A. Coleman — *Editor*
Robin Fitzpatrick Husayko — *Editor*
Dorothy A. Johnson — *Editorial Assistant*

AMA CONSULTING BOARD

Bruce Berkson, MD
Urology

Steven N. Blair, PhD
Epidemiology/Fitness

Richard C. Bozian, MD
Nutrition

Rowland W. Chang, MD
Rheumatology

Melvin Cheitlin, MD
Cardiology

Priscilla M. Clarkson, PhD
Physiology

Joseph L. Clayman, MD
Dermatology

Bruce Cohen, MD
Neurology

David Cugell, MD
Pulmonary Medicine

Raymond H. Curry, MD
Internal Medicine

Arthur W. Curtis, MD
Otolaryngology

Kimberly A. Douglass, RN
Clinical Nurse Specialist

Richard M. Gore, MD
Radiology

Jourdan Gottlieb, MD
Plastic and Reconstructive Surgery

Donald F. Heiman, MD
Infectious Diseases

Linda Hughey Holt, MD
Obstetrics and Gynecology

Allen Horwitz, MD
Genetics

Howard N. Jacobson, MD
Nutrition

Frederic C. Kass, MD
Oncology

Robert J. Kelsey, Jr., MD
Obstetrics and Gynecology

Gary S. Lissner, MD
Ophthalmology

Kenneth R. Margules, MD
Rheumatology

Mary Ann McCann
Pharmacology/Toxicology

Arline McDonald, PhD
Nutrition

Ronald M. Meyer, MD
Anesthesiology

Gary Noskin, MD
Infectious Diseases

Robert V. Rege, MD
General Surgery

Domeena C. Renshaw, MD
Psychiatry/Sexual Dysfunction

Gary A. Rodgers, DDS
Dentistry

Andrew T. Saltzman, MD
Orthopedics

Mary Beth Shwayder, MD
Pathology

Michael W. T. Shwayder, MD
Nephrology

Irwin M. Siegel, MD
Orthopedics

Emanuel M. Steindler
Addiction Medicine

Mark Stolar, MD
Endocrinology

Ronald J. Vasu, MD
Psychiatry

DORLING KINDERSLEY

Editorial Director Jonathan Reed; **Series Editor** Robert Dinwiddie; **Senior Editor** Andrea Bagg
Editors Amanda Jackson, Gail Lawther, Maxine Lewis, Caroline Macy, Dr. Fiona Payne, Joanna Thomas
Production Manager Ian Paton; **Production Editor** Edda Bohnsack; **Production Assistant** Margaret Little
Design Director Ed Day; **Series Art Editor** Simon Webb; **Art Editor** Mark Batley
Designers Amanda Carroll, Yaël Freudmann, Jenny Howley, Lydia Umney, Virginia Walter
Picture Research Julia Tacey

CONTENTS

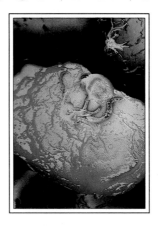

CHAPTER ONE

A WORLD OF MICROBES

WE LIVE IN A SEA OF GERMS. As a result, we are constantly waging war against these microscopic disease organisms, called microorganisms or microbes. For the most part, our bodies successfully defend us. A very small number of microbes – called pathogens – consistently cause disease. Most microorganisms become infectious only when the body's defenses break down. Pathogens include a variety of tiny life-forms – mainly bacteria, viruses, and fungi – and parasites such as worms and lice that infest the body. Our potential enemies range from simple structures that are little bigger than large molecules, to tapeworms, which are highly complex organisms that contain a set of both male and female reproductive organs and can grow to 20 feet. Millions of bacteria permanently inhabit the skin and the mucous membranes that line the mouth, nose, intestines, and vagina. These organisms act as barriers that protect us from dangerous invading microorganisms. They do so by using all the available nutritional resources the invaders would otherwise depend on for nourishment. But sometimes these usually beneficial organisms or the invading germs manage to penetrate the protective mucous membranes and travel into internal tissues.

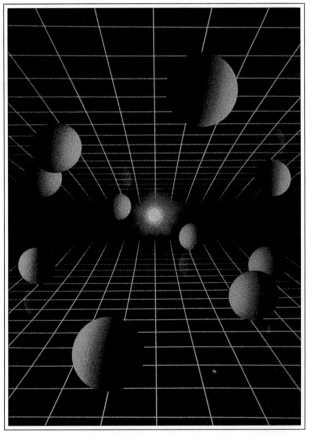

When they do so, they can cause infections. Infectious diseases present much less of a threat in technologically advanced countries today than they did in the early years of this century. Many serious diseases, such as diphtheria and polio, have been virtually eliminated through immunization programs. Major scourges associated with bacterial infections – notably rheumatic and scarlet fevers – have become rare with improvements in nutrition and the use of antibiotics to treat them. In the US, the three infections that require quarantine – cholera, yellow fever, and plague – are all extremely rare. Other illnesses, such as typhoid fever, caused many deaths in the early part of this century but have gradually diminished. Pneumococcal pneumonia, a serious form of pneumonia, is still common but can be treated with antibiotics. The decline of many infectious diseases has resulted from a combination of the use of effective vaccines and antibiotics, and safe water and sewage systems.

In this chapter, we review the wide range of disease organisms, how they are transmitted, and how our bodies respond to them. Later sections explore the history of the fight against infections and the course of epidemics, and review the groups of infectious diseases that occur in the US today.

WHAT IS AN INFECTION ?

Our bodies swarm with many types of harmless microscopic organisms, called microorganisms or microbes. It is only when these friendly organisms (or harmful ones) penetrate natural barriers such as the mucous membranes and multiply that we experience the symptoms of an infection. Symptoms such as a fever are the result of the body's response to disease organisms. An infection may be present in one part of the body or throughout it.

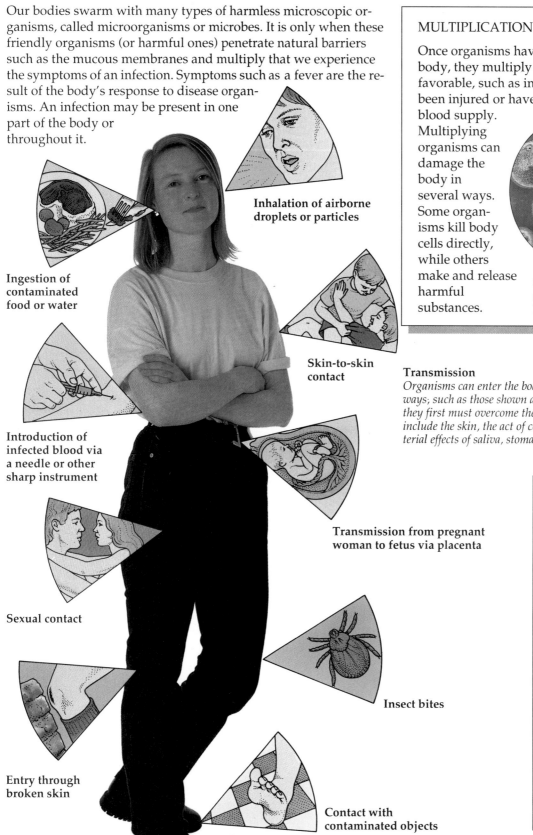

Inhalation of airborne droplets or particles

Ingestion of contaminated food or water

Skin-to-skin contact

Introduction of infected blood via a needle or other sharp instrument

Transmission from pregnant woman to fetus via placenta

Sexual contact

Insect bites

Entry through broken skin

Contact with contaminated objects

MULTIPLICATION

Once organisms have entered the body, they multiply if conditions are favorable, such as in tissues that have been injured or have an impaired blood supply. Multiplying organisms can damage the body in several ways. Some organisms kill body cells directly, while others make and release harmful substances.

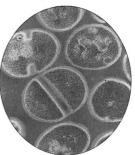

Staphylococcus aureus **(magnified 18,500 times)**

Transmission

Organisms can enter the body in many different ways; such as those shown at left. To cause infection, they first must overcome the body's barriers, which include the skin, the act of coughing, or the antibacterial effects of saliva, stomach acid, and tears.

INCUBATION PERIOD

The incubation period of an infectious disease is the time between a person's exposure to the disease organism and the development of the first symptoms. Most infectious diseases have a consistent, defined incubation period. For example, almost every child will break out in the characteristic rash of chickenpox within 2 or 3 weeks after he or she has been exposed to the virus.

LOCAL INFECTIONS

In local infections, the disease-causing organisms remain in one part of the body. Local infections range from minor or annoying disorders, such as an infected hangnail or outer-ear infection (shown here), to potentially life-threatening conditions, such as pneumonia.

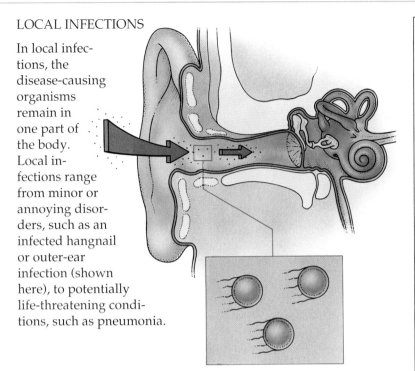

IMMUNE SYSTEM RESPONSE

The immune system is a group of cells and proteins that can recognize the presence of foreign proteins (antigens) and respond to eliminate the invaders. Once a person has been infected by a specific germ, an immune response is stimulated to protect against future infections by the same organism. Without previous exposure, the body's response is slower and illness is more likely. Many symptoms of an infection are the result of the struggle between the body's defenses and the disease organisms.

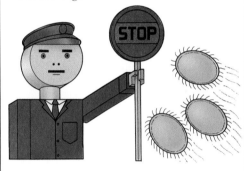

INFLAMMATORY RESPONSE

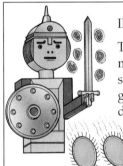

The response to a local infection is inflammation, characterized by redness, heat, swelling, and pain. Inflammation is triggered by chemical substances released by disease organisms and by body cells that have been damaged. The chemicals attract white blood cells to the site to combat the invading microbes.

LATENT INFECTIONS

Some infections remain dormant in the body, apparently causing no harm, for months or years. In untreated syphilis, for example, there are very few symptoms during the first stage. After the first stage, weeks or months may pass without any signs before the rashes of the second stage appear and then disappear. The symptoms of the dangerous third stage may not develop for several years.

SYSTEMIC INFECTIONS

Sometimes, disease organisms and/or their toxins travel throughout the body, causing widespread (systemic) infections. Symptoms may include a fever, rash, and aches and pains. Chickenpox is a familiar systemic infection.

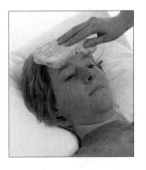

Rash
Rashes often accompany systemic infections. A rash – one or more areas of inflamed skin – frequently causes itching.

Fever
Fever occurs when substances released by defensive white blood cells reset the body's thermostat in the brain to a higher level.

OUTCOME OF INFECTION

The outcome of an infection depends on three main factors – the virulence (harmfulness) of the invading organism, the number of organisms present, and the response of the immune system. The efficiency of the immune system is crucial. A healthy immune system can cope well with most infections. A compromised immune system, as a result of diseases such as cancer or AIDS, may allow usually harmless organisms to proliferate and cause widespread, serious disease.

INFECTIOUS AGENTS

Disease organisms vary from tiny viruses to 20-foot-long tapeworms. All the organisms illustrated on this page are color enhanced and drawn to the same scale – 7,000 times their actual size. The worm larva, which is only about 0.008 inch long, is so large compared with the other organisms that only the tip can be shown. Individual magnifications are given for the photographs, which are not depicted to the same scale.

PROTOZOA
Protozoa are single-celled animals that cause some diarrheal illnesses; trichomoniasis (a sexually transmitted infection); and toxoplasmosis, which is acquired by eating undercooked meat or by contact with feces of infected cats or birds.

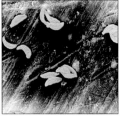

Toxoplasma gondii
(protozoan; causes toxoplasmosis; magnified 800 times)

Poliovirus

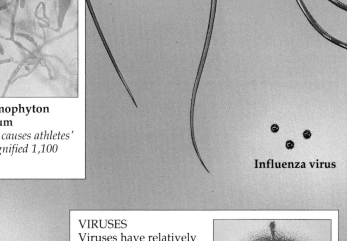

Giardia lamblia (protozoan; causes giardiasis, an intestinal infection)

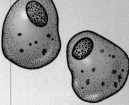

Plasmodium vivax (protozoan; causes one type of malaria)

FUNGI
Fungi are simple, parasitic life-forms that may grow into colonies of individual cells or branched chains of cells. Fungal diseases include ringworm (a skin infection), candidiasis (commonly known as a yeast infection), and histoplasmosis (a serious lung disease).

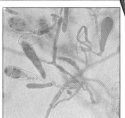

Epidermophyton floccosum
(fungus; causes athletes' foot; magnified 1,100 times)

Influenza virus

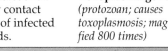

Rabies virus

VIRUSES
Viruses have relatively simple structures. They can multiply only after they have invaded the cells of other life-forms. Viruses cause colds, influenza, measles, AIDS, rabies, warts, cold sores, polio, and many cases of gastroenteritis (inflammation of the stomach and intestines).

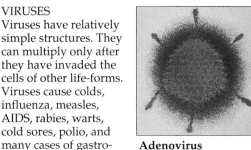

Adenovirus
(causes colds and sore throats; magnified 38,100 times)

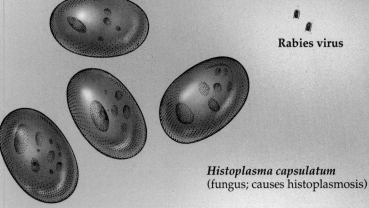

Histoplasma capsulatum (fungus; causes histoplasmosis)

Rickettsia rickettsii (bacterium; causes Rocky Mountain spotted fever, a disease transmitted by tick bites)

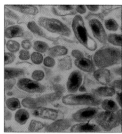

Coxiella burnetii *(rickettsia bacterium; causes Q fever; magnified 16,800 times)*

CHLAMYDIAE AND RICKETTSIAE
Chlamydiae are a group of small bacteria that cause genital, eye, and lung infections. Infections caused by another group of small bacteria, called rickettsiae, include Q fever (an illness that affects the respiratory system) and Rocky Mountain spotted fever.

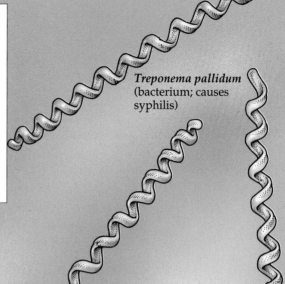

Treponema pallidum (bacterium; causes syphilis)

Herpesvirus

BACTERIA
Bacteria come in various shapes including spheres (cocci), rods (bacilli), and spirals (spirochetes). Boils, salmonellosis (a type of food poisoning), gonorrhea, syphilis, tuberculosis, and many cases of sore throat are caused by bacteria.

Clostridium botulinum *(bacterium; causes food poisoning; magnified 1,300 times)*

Chlamydia trachomatis (bacterium; causes eye and genital infections)

HIV (human immunodeficiency virus; causes AIDS)

HELMINTHS (WORMS)
This group of parasites includes roundworms, which have cylindrical bodies, and flatworms, such as tapeworms and flukes. Worm diseases include infestations with pinworms and hookworms, and toxocariasis (infestation with a worm larva).

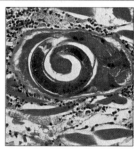

Trichinella spiralis *(acquired by eating undercooked pork; causes trichinosis; magnified 50 times)*

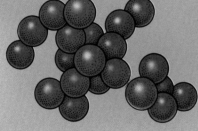

Staphylococcus aureus (bacterium; causes boils and other infections)

Campylobacter jejuni (bacterium; causes gastroenteritis)

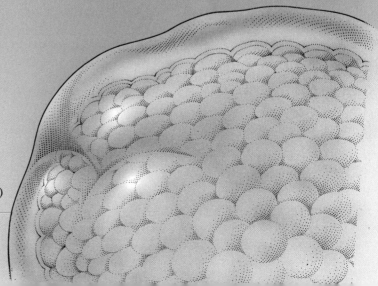

Toxocara canis (worm larva; causes toxocariasis)

HOW INFECTIONS ARE TRANSMITTED

Most people who acquire an infection have had direct contact with an infected person or have been exposed to germs that have contaminated air, soil, water, or food. Less frequently, infections are acquired from animals (see page 16). Some illnesses occur after an invasion by only a few disease organisms. For other infections, up to a million organisms may be required to cause illness. You should be aware of the ways in which infectious diseases are transmitted (see below) and take precautions to avoid them.

(see page 16)

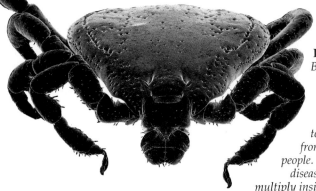

Insect bites
Bloodsucking insects can spread infections from person to person and from animals to people. Usually, the disease organisms multiply inside the insect and are passed on when the insect bites a person. Mosquitoes spread malaria and epidemic encephalitis. Ticks (such as the one shown here, magnified 18 times) spread Lyme disease and Rocky Mountain spotted fever.

PREVENTING INFECTIONS

You can avoid many infections by following these simple rules:

◆ When possible, stay away from anyone with a respiratory infection. Teach your children to cover their mouths and noses with a tissue when they sneeze or cough.

◆ Avoid hand contact with anyone who has a respiratory infection.

◆ Wash your hands regularly with soap and water, particularly before meals and after using the toilet. Keep your hands away from your mouth.

◆ Do not pick at blemishes on your skin; you may spread an infection to other areas.

◆ Thoroughly clean and cover cuts and wounds. All serious cuts and all animal or human bites require medical attention.

◆ Avoid eating in places that have noticeably poor standards of hygiene.

Skin-to-skin contact
Most organisms cannot penetrate the skin. However, some staphylococcal bacteria cause boils and some streptococcal bacteria can cause skin infections such as impetigo, which usually occurs around the nose and mouth. Fungal skin diseases such as ringworm (shown right) and viral skin diseases such as genital warts and herpes simplex infections (which cause cold sores) can also be spread by skin-to-skin contact.

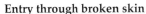

Blood transfusions
AIDS, hepatitis B and C, and syphilis can be spread through transfusions with infected blood or blood products. Screening blood donors and testing blood have made transfusion-related infections rare today.

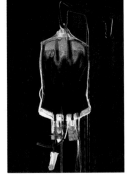

Entry through broken skin
Many infectious organisms can enter the body through a break in the skin. Spores of the bacterium Clostridium tetani, which live mainly in soil and manure, can enter a person's body through a cut or puncture wound. Such an invasion causes tetanus, a serious condition that can lead to nervous system damage.

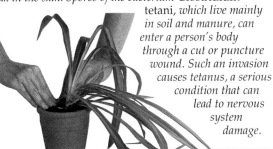

Self-contamination of the eye, nose, or mouth
Viral respiratory infections, such as colds, are often acquired by direct contact, such as shaking hands with an infected person. These infections can also be spread when people touch their eyes, nose, or mouth after touching a contaminated object. The infectious organisms enter the body through the mucous membranes.

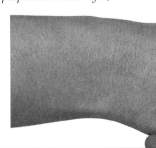

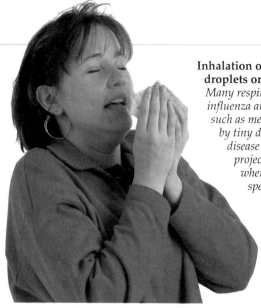

Inhalation of airborne droplets or particles

Many respiratory infections (including influenza and pneumonia) and other diseases such as meningitis and measles are spread by tiny droplets of liquid containing disease organisms. An infected person projects these droplets into the air when he or she coughs, sneezes, or speaks. Another person may then inhale the airborne infectious droplets. Sometimes disease organisms, such as those that cause the fungal lung infection histoplasmosis, are inhaled directly or as contaminants on dust particles.

Introduction of infected blood via a needle or other sharp instrument

Some infecting organisms, such as those that cause viral hepatitis types B and C and AIDS, are present in blood and can be transmitted from an infected person to a healthy person by blood-to-blood contact. This contact most commonly occurs when users of illegal drugs share needles, but can also happen during tattooing, acupuncture, ear piercing, or dental and surgical procedures.

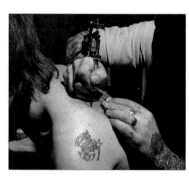

Ingestion of contaminated food or water

Some illnesses, such as viral hepatitis type A (an infection of the liver) and intestinal infections such as salmonella food poisoning, are spread when organisms present in an infected person's feces contaminate food or drinking water. The transmission of germs usually occurs when an infected person fails to wash his or her hands after using the toilet and then touches food being prepared for others. Drinking water can become contaminated as a result of inadequate water purification or sewage disposal.

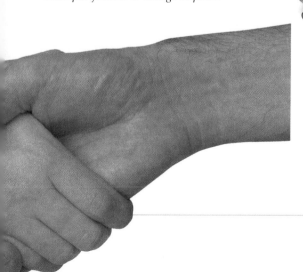

Sexual contact

Some disease organisms – such as those that cause viral hepatitis types B and C, AIDS, and syphilis – may be 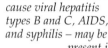 *present in semen or in vaginal secretions. These disease organisms can enter the body through the mucous membranes of the vagina, anus, and mouth during sexual contact. Infections of the mucous membranes – such as genital herpes, gonorrhea, and candidiasis – and infestations with crab lice are also transmitted by sexual contact.*

CARRIERS OF INFECTION

Most people who spread an infectious disease have obvious signs and symptoms. However, people can be carriers of disease-causing organisms and not know it because they do not experience any symptoms of illness. The infectious organisms reproduce in the carrier's body and can be passed on to others. Organisms commonly transmitted by apparently healthy carriers include those that cause trichomoniasis, AIDS, and viral hepatitis types B and C.

Trichomoniasis

Trichomoniasis is a mild, but very common, sexually transmitted disease that is caused by a protozoan. The infection can cause genital pain and irritation. Most infected men have no symptoms but can spread the disease to their sexual partners.

HIV carriers

A person may be infected with HIV (human immunodeficiency virus, which causes AIDS) and not have any symptoms for several years. The AIDS virus can be transmitted through blood-to-blood contact and exposure to other body fluids such as those exchanged during sexual contact.

Long-term, contagious disease

A person may have an infectious disease for a long time, without appearing seriously ill, but still be highly infectious. In some cases of hepatitis B, for instance, an infected person may recover from the actual illness, but still carry the virus in his or her bloodstream. A pregnant woman who is a hepatitis B carrier can infect her baby at birth. Babies who acquire hepatitis B at birth are much more likely to become chronic carriers of the virus than are people who become infected at older ages.

DISEASES ACQUIRED FROM ANIMALS

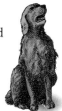

Some diseases that are common in animals can also infect people. In urban areas, few diseases are spread to people from animals. But some that are – such as toxoplasmosis (transmitted by cats), toxocariasis (transmitted by cats and dogs), and psittacosis (transmitted by birds) – can cause serious illness. Farm animals are sources of a number of infections that can be transmitted to humans, either directly or through consumption of contaminated meat or milk. Wild animals also carry many diseases. They are still a significant source of disease in developing countries, but pose less risk of infection to people in the US and other developed countries.

HOW DOES TRANSMISSION OCCUR?

A variety of disease-causing organisms can be passed from animals to people in many ways.

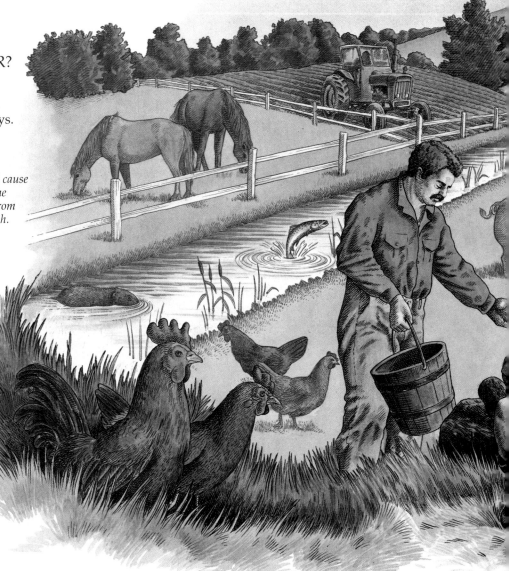

Tapeworms
Tapeworms invade the intestines and cause intestinal disorders. People acquire the worms by eating undercooked meat from an infected pig, cow, or freshwater fish.

Plague
Rodents carry this serious but rare bacterial infection, which is transmitted to people by bites from infected fleas.

Leptospirosis
This bacterial infection, which is transmitted through contact with the urine of infected rodents and domestic animals such as dogs, can cause severe illness in people. Swimming in contaminated water may also lead to infection.

Brucellosis
Contact with infected farm animals causes this bacterial infection, which poses a hazard for farm and slaughterhouse workers. Nonpasteurized milk is another source of brucellosis.

Toxocariasis
This relatively rare condition can cause inflammation of many organ systems, including the eye. Worms normally present in dogs and cats are transmitters of the infection. Worm eggs in the animals' feces often contaminate soil, posing a risk for children who play with the soil and then put their hands in their mouths.

Salmonellosis
This serious infection can develop when a person eats food, particularly poultry and eggs, that is contaminated with salmonella bacteria.

Psittacosis
Inhaling chlamydia bacteria from the dried dust of bird droppings causes this serious lung infection.

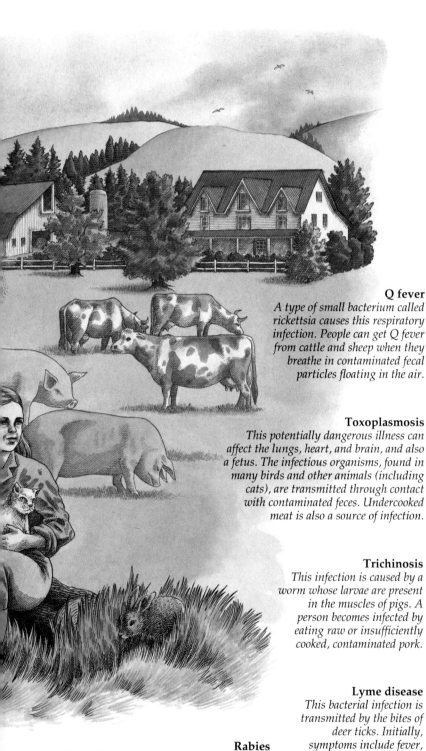

Q fever

A type of small bacterium called rickettsia causes this respiratory infection. People can get Q fever from cattle and sheep when they breathe in contaminated fecal particles floating in the air.

Toxoplasmosis

This potentially dangerous illness can affect the lungs, heart, and brain, and also a fetus. The infectious organisms, found in many birds and other animals (including cats), are transmitted through contact with contaminated feces. Undercooked meat is also a source of infection.

Trichinosis

This infection is caused by a worm whose larvae are present in the muscles of pigs. A person becomes infected by eating raw or insufficiently cooked, contaminated pork.

Lyme disease

This bacterial infection is transmitted by the bites of deer ticks. Initially, symptoms include fever, chills, muscle aches, and a rash. When not treated, Lyme disease can lead to complications affecting the brain, heart, and joints.

Rabies

This acute viral infection of the nervous system is transmitted by an infected animal that bites someone or licks a person's broken skin.

Rocky Mountain spotted fever

This infectious disease is caused by a rickettsia bacterium. It is transmitted from small mammals to people by tick bites.

AVOIDING INFECTIONS FROM PETS

Follow these guidelines to avoid getting infections from your pets:

◆ Regularly change the litter in cat litter boxes and clean out bird cages and the living quarters of any pets; wear gloves. Wash your hands well when you are finished. Avoid inhaling dust from litter boxes, cages, and rabbit hutches.

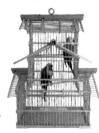

◆ If your cat scratches you, wash the area thoroughly and cover it with a bandage. If you are bitten or severely scratched by an animal, clean the wound well, cover it with a bandage, and see your doctor. You may need to take medication.

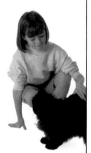

◆ Have your pets checked regularly by a veterinarian; cats and dogs require routine vaccinations and preventive treatment against parasites and infections.

◆ Discourage your pets from defecating in your yard. Provide a litter tray for your cat and walk your dog regularly. Clean up any feces in the house immediately and disinfect the area.

◆ Teach your children to wash their hands after playing outside and to avoid putting their hands in or around their mouths when they are dirty.

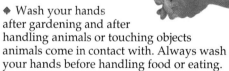

◆ Wash your hands after gardening and after handling animals or touching objects animals come in contact with. Always wash your hands before handling food or eating.

◆ Do not use the same food dishes for people and animals. Wash animal food bowls separately.

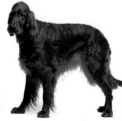

◆ Don't allow pets to lick you on the mouth.

INFECTION DURING PREGNANCY AND CHILDBIRTH

During pregnancy, the placenta links the blood supplies of the pregnant woman and fetus. Their blood does not actually mix, but the placenta conveys nutrients and oxygen to the fetus and removes waste products. Many infectious organisms can pass across the placenta to the fetus in this way (see right and below). Some infections – such as gonorrhea, herpes, and streptococcal infections – can be acquired by the baby during delivery through contact with disease organisms present in the birth canal.

How disease organisms reach the fetus
In the placenta, fetal blood vessels are surrounded by maternal blood, allowing substances such as nutrients to pass easily from the mother's blood to the fetus's blood. While the placenta blocks the passage of most harmful substances, some disease organisms can reach the fetus. These include organisms that cause chickenpox, toxoplasmosis, cytomegalovirus, syphilis, AIDS, and rubella.

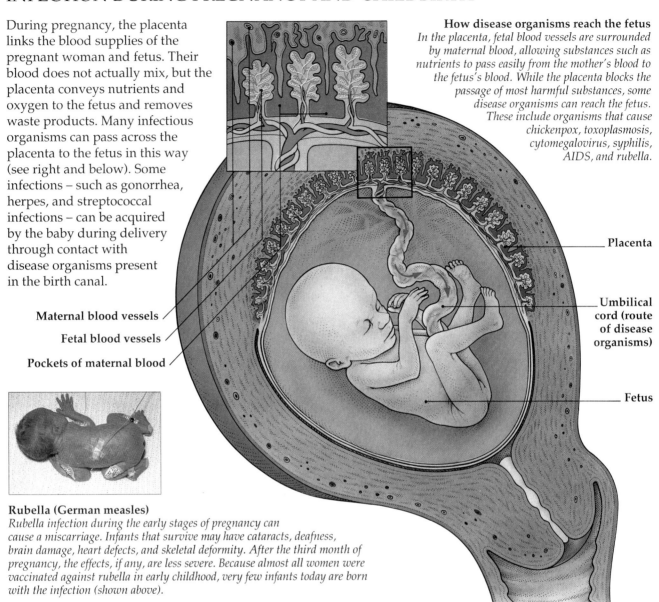

Maternal blood vessels
Fetal blood vessels
Pockets of maternal blood

Placenta

Umbilical cord (route of disease organisms)

Fetus

Rubella (German measles)
Rubella infection during the early stages of pregnancy can cause a miscarriage. Infants that survive may have cataracts, deafness, brain damage, heart defects, and skeletal deformity. After the third month of pregnancy, the effects, if any, are less severe. Because almost all women were vaccinated against rubella in early childhood, very few infants today are born with the infection (shown above).

EFFECTS OF INFECTIONS ON THE FETUS

Some infectious diseases acquired by a fetus during pregnancy can be extremely serious.

◆ Herpes simplex virus is usually transmitted to a fetus during delivery through an infected woman's genital tract. In these cases, doctors may perform a cesarean section to avoid passage through the birth canal. An active herpes infection during pregnancy may lead to miscarriage, premature labor, or birth defects.

◆ Toxoplasmosis, particularly if acquired by a woman in the second trimester of pregnancy, may be life-threatening to a fetus. If the fetus survives, he or she may have severe eye defects and mental retardation.

◆ Cytomegalovirus (a member of the herpesvirus family) may cause a baby to be mentally retarded and to have hearing problems. Most babies have no ill effects.

◆ AIDS is caused by HIV (human immunodeficiency virus), which infects about one third of the babies born to women with AIDS.

◆ Syphilis, transmitted from an infected pregnant woman to her fetus, increases the risks of stillbirth, newborn death, or birth defects. Congenital (present at birth) syphilis, which is on the rise in the US, can usually be prevented by treating the woman during the first trimester of pregnancy.

FEATURES OF INFECTION

The course an infection takes depends on several factors – the number and nature of the infecting organisms, their ability to cause disease, where they enter the body and how they spread through it, and the speed and effectiveness of the body's response to them. An organism's ability to cause severe illness – its virulence – depends on how easily it is transmitted and on how successfully it invades body tissues once the infection has taken hold. A virulent strain of influenza can make a third or more of the exposed population very ill; a less virulent strain may infect fewer people and cause fewer and less severe symptoms in those who are infected.

Spread within the body

Most disease organisms do not get far into the body. They are halted by an inflammatory response to their presence

MECHANISMS OF MULTIPLICATION

Disease organisms multiply under favorable conditions – the right temperature, enough moisture, a supply of nutrients, and, in the case of viruses, suitable body cells in which to multiply. Different organisms have different methods of multiplication.

Bacteria
multiply by dividing into two cells, which, in turn, divide. Under optimum conditions, colonies of bacteria can double in size every 20 minutes.

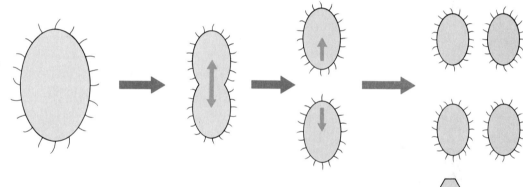

Viruses
hijack the chemical machinery of body cells to make copies of themselves. As with other organisms, many viruses selectively invade specific organs or tissues in which they are able to multiply.

Virus   └ Body cell

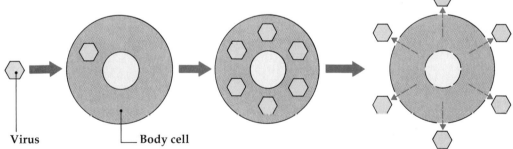

Protozoa
reproduce in different ways. Some multiply by splitting into two (binary fission), while others divide into several daughter parasites (schizogony). Some protozoa exist in male and female forms and multiply sexually.

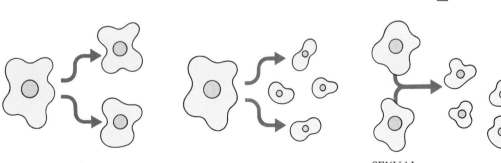

BINARY FISSION   SCHIZOGONY   SEXUAL REPRODUCTION

19

(see INFLAMMATORY RESPONSE on page 21). The invading organisms usually cause limited infections confined to one area of the body. Some organisms spread through the lymphatic system, an important part of the body's defenses. When the invaders reach a lymph node, they are attacked by lymphocytes, which are a type of white blood cell. This defensive response may result in swelling of the nodes. In other cases, organisms may gain access to the bloodstream, potentially causing a life-threatening infection that affects the whole body.

HARMFUL EFFECTS

Viruses cause disease by disrupting the functioning of body cells or by killing them directly. Viral infections commonly cause high fever, muscle pain, headache, and loss of energy. These

Swollen glands
The spread of organisms to lymph nodes (also called lymph glands) may cause the nodes to swell. For example, if you have an infection in your arm or throat, you may notice swelling in the lymph nodes of your armpit or neck.

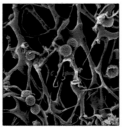

Lymphocytes
The illustration above shows the presence of lymphocytes (which appear as spherical cells) inside a lymph node.

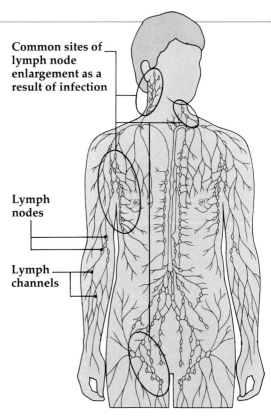

Common sites of lymph node enlargement as a result of infection

Lymph nodes

Lymph channels

HARMFUL EFFECTS OF BACTERIAL TOXINS

Bacteria cause much of their damage by manufacturing toxins (poisons) and releasing them into the body.

1 Bacterial toxins may interfere with normal chemical reactions in cells, killing the cells or preventing them from functioning.

Bacteria   **Body cells**

Toxins

Damaged or dead cells

2 Toxins may cause blood to clot in small vessels, blocking them and causing damage to areas deprived of blood.

Bacteria

Toxins

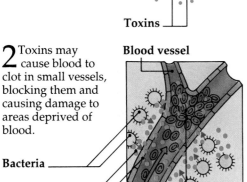

Blood vessel

Blood clot

Area of tissue deprived of blood and damaged

3 Toxins can damage the walls of small vessels, causing them to leak. When too much fluid is lost from the circulation, the heart is unable to maintain an adequate blood supply to the brain and to its own muscular wall.

Toxins   **Blood vessel**

Gaps appear between cells in blood vessel wall

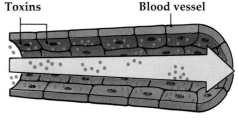

Fluid leaks into tissues   **Toxins**

INFLAMMATORY RESPONSE

Inflammation is the body's response to a local infection; one of the major purposes of inflammation is to contain an infection.

1 Release of bacterial toxins and the body's response to infection damage cells. As a result of this damage, inflammatory substances are released into the blood, provoking reactions in local blood vessels.

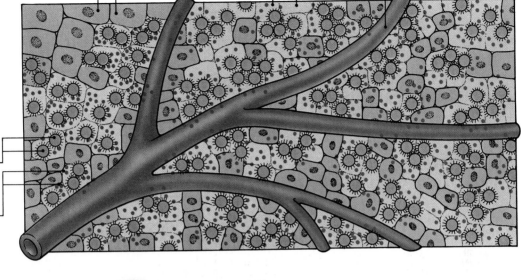

Body cells — Damaged body cells — Blood vessel

Disease organisms —

Inflammatory substances —

2 In response to the release of inflammatory substances (including histamine and prostaglandins) the blood vessels widen and leak, and blood flow increases. These processes cause redness, heat, and swelling. The inflammatory substances also stimulate nerve endings, causing pain.

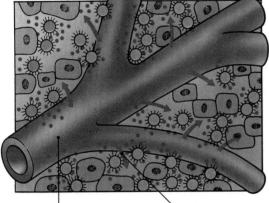

Widened blood vessel — Escaping fluid

4 Some bacteria respond by producing toxins that destroy defensive white blood cells. The debris of the conflict – destroyed bacteria, destroyed white blood cells, and damaged cells – accumulates as pus. Sometimes the body forms a protective membrane around the site, creating an abscess.

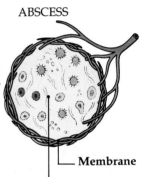

ABSCESS

— Membrane

Pus formed from dead cells and organisms

Blood vessel — Phagocyte

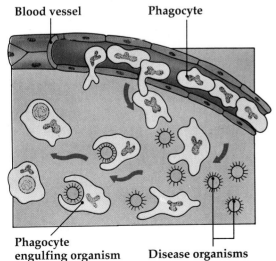

Phagocyte engulfing organism — Disease organisms

3 Bacterial toxins and chemical messengers released from damaged tissue attract white blood cells called phagocytes to the site of infection. The phagocytes clump together and squeeze through the blood vessel walls to engulf and destroy the invaders.

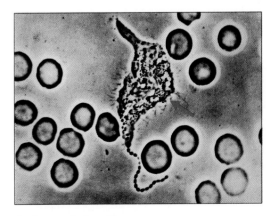

A phagocyte in action
The photograph above (magnified 1,400 times) shows a phagocyte (arrow) ingesting a chain of streptococcal bacteria. The round objects are red blood cells.

21

RASHES

Rashes, a common characteristic of infections affecting the whole body, usually fall into one of three categories represented by the infections shown at right. Few rashes uniformly cover the body. The appearance of the individual spots and their distribution is often enough for a doctor to diagnose the illness. Diseases produce rashes as individual as fingerprints. Many rashes can also result from allergic reactions to drugs.

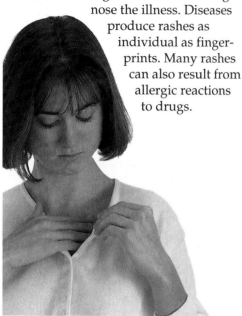

Measles
Rashes with flat or slightly raised reddish spots, or combinations of the two, occur in measles (shown at left). Many viral infections, typhoid fever, and the second stage of syphilis also have this type of rash.

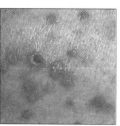

Chickenpox
Sometimes rashes have raised swellings that contain fluid. The fluid may be either clear (as in blisters) or consist of pus. Chickenpox (shown at left), herpes (cold sores), shingles (a reactivation of the chickenpox virus), and several other viral infections have rashes with blisters.

Blood poisoning
Bleeding into the skin causes purpuric rashes, which take the form of tiny, dark, purplish spots. Infections that produce purpuric rashes include a type of blood poisoning (shown at right) and Rocky Mountain spotted fever.

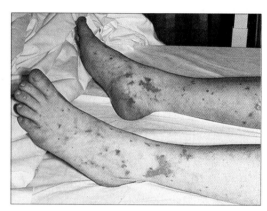

symptoms are in part the result of the effects of powerful proteins produced by the body to fight the infection.

Bacteria cause disease by killing cells and by producing potent toxins (see HARMFUL EFFECTS OF BACTERIAL TOXINS on page 20). Bacteria can get into the bloodstream and circulate throughout the body, multiplying and producing toxins that cause a serious reaction. Victims of such blood poisoning have a high fever and chills and feel very weak.

Blood poisoning may progress to an even more dangerous condition – septic shock, in which there is tissue damage and a dramatic drop in blood pressure. Septic shock requires immediate medical treatment, which includes intravenous antibiotic drugs and measures to maintain blood volume and pressure. Surgery to remove the source of infection – such as an infected gallbladder or appendix – may be necessary.

IMMUNE SYSTEM RESPONSE

The responsiveness of the immune system has a marked effect on the course of an infection. Many types of white blood cells and antibodies play a role (see THE BODY'S DEFENSES on page 62). White blood cells called B lymphocytes produce antibodies that circulate and attack specific invading organisms. The invaders are then easy targets for other white blood cells called phagocytes, which engulf and destroy them.

When a person's immune system has been "primed" by infection with a specific organism, it is able to respond quickly to subsequent infections by the same organism. Without previous exposure, the immune system may take several days or weeks to eliminate the infection. The person may become severely ill.

FEVER
During an infection, a substance called interleukin-1, released by white blood cells called phagocytes, resets the body's natural thermostat in the brain to a higher level. As a result, the brain signals the body to increase heat production, causing symptoms, such as uncontrollable shivering, that help to raise the temperature. When infectious organisms are multiplying in the bloodstream, the body temperature may reach as high as 104°F.

OPPORTUNISTIC INFECTIONS

In opportunistic infections, organisms cause disease by taking advantage of a reduction in the efficiency of a person's immune system. The immune system may be suppressed in various ways, including treatment with corticosteroid and anticancer drugs and long-term antibiotic therapy. Certain diseases, such as leukemia, AIDS, and diabetes, also cause reduced immunity and make a person more susceptible to infection.

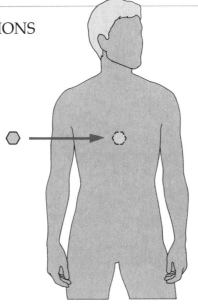

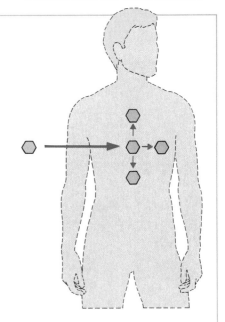

Healthy immune system
In a person with a healthy immune system, many potentially harmful organisms are quickly attacked by the body's defenses, almost always preventing infection.

Weakened immune system
In a person with a weakened immune system, organisms that are usually harmless may thrive and spread freely, causing severe infection.

OUTCOME

Many factors influence the effectiveness of the immune response and, therefore, the outcome of an infection. A person who is severely malnourished, because of factors such as a poor diet or alcoholism, may not form enough antibodies to successfully fight an infection.

Barriers to infection, such as the skin and the immune system, may be compromised by certain medical conditions. A badly burned person, or someone with severe eczema (a skin condition that can cause scaling and blistering), loses the protection of the intact skin. Anticancer drugs may interfere with the action of the defensive white blood cells, resulting in an insufficient immune response. Smoking can hinder the lungs' natural defenses and the efficient functioning of the immune system.

In addition, individuals vary in their susceptibility to infection. Some people are born with a relative inability to produce antibodies. Other inherited factors may also help determine the effectiveness of a person's immune response.

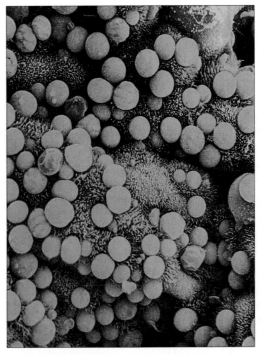

Cryptosporidiosis
The color-enhanced photograph above shows large numbers of the protozoal parasite Cryptosporidium parvum *(green spheres; magnified 1,500 times) in the intestine of a person with AIDS. Cryptosporidiosis is a common opportunistic infection that is a frequent cause of death in people who have AIDS. Pneumocystis pneumonia, various fungal infections, and severe infections with herpesviruses, including cytomegalovirus, are other common opportunistic infections.*

LETHALITY

Lethality is the ability of a disease to cause death. Chickenpox has a very low lethality, while AIDS probably has a 100 percent lethality – it is fatal for everyone who gets it. Often, the lethality of an organism depends on the susceptibility of the people exposed to it. Measles is a mild or moderate illness in populations in which it commonly occurs because many people have developed some immunity through exposure to the infection. But measles introduced for the first time into a population with no immunity can cause an epidemic with a significant death rate.

POPULATIONS AND INFECTIONS

Infectious organisms spread through a population with varying degrees of success. Among the important factors necessary for an infection to take hold and spread are the number of organisms required to cause illness, the disease's mode of transmission, and the number of people who are naturally immune to or have been vaccinated against it.

EPIDEMICS

A sudden, large-scale increase in the number of cases of an infectious disease within a population is called an epidemic. An epidemic occurs when a disease organism is introduced into a population that has a large number of people who are susceptible to infection by that organism. A weakened immune system or lack of immunity to the disease organism can make a person vulnerable.

Natural disasters such as earthquakes can cause epidemics by disrupting public water supplies and sewage systems. People may then be exposed to water that is contaminated with bacteria and other disease-causing organisms.

ENDEMIC DISEASES

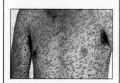

A disease is said to be endemic in a population when the population always includes at least some people who have the disease. The infection never completely dies out within that population. Diseases that are endemic in most populations include chickenpox (shown above), viral infections of the upper respiratory tract (colds), infectious mononucleosis, staphylococcal and streptococcal skin diseases, meningitis, and streptococcal throat infections.

KEY

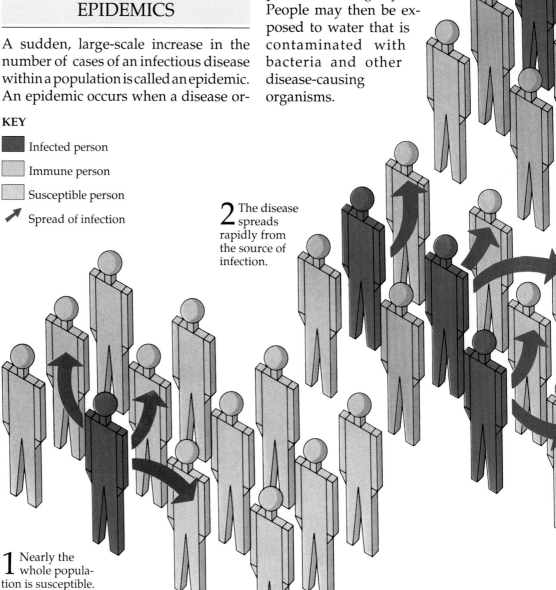

- ■ Infected person
- ▢ Immune person
- ▢ Susceptible person
- ➚ Spread of infection

2 The disease spreads rapidly from the source of infection.

1 Nearly the whole population is susceptible.

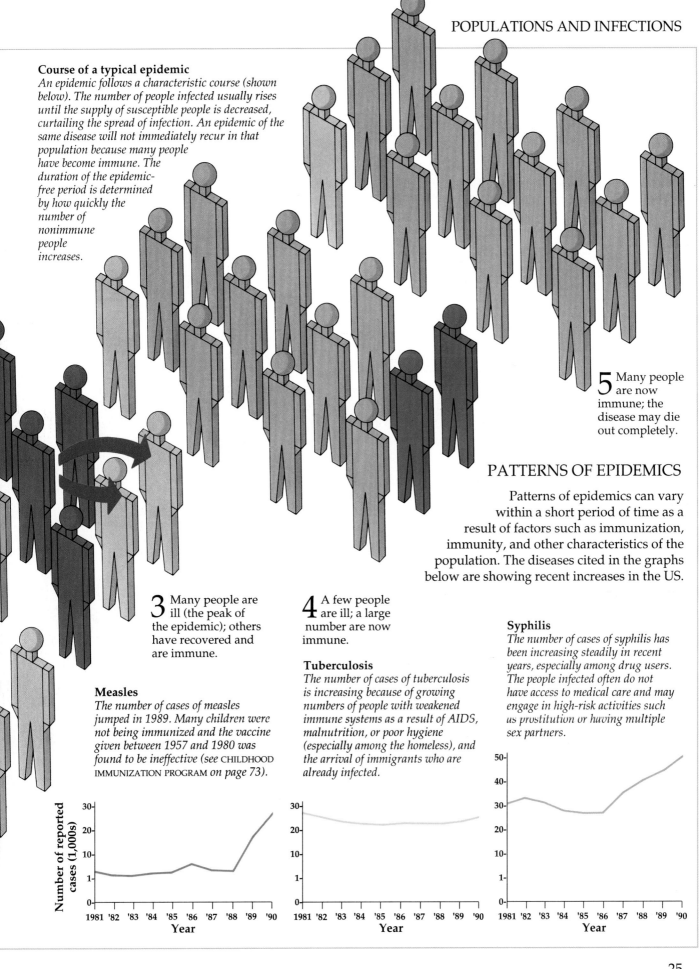

Course of a typical epidemic
An epidemic follows a characteristic course (shown below). The number of people infected usually rises until the supply of susceptible people is decreased, curtailing the spread of infection. An epidemic of the same disease will not immediately recur in that population because many people have become immune. The duration of the epidemic-free period is determined by how quickly the number of nonimmune people increases.

5 Many people are now immune; the disease may die out completely.

PATTERNS OF EPIDEMICS

Patterns of epidemics can vary within a short period of time as a result of factors such as immunization, immunity, and other characteristics of the population. The diseases cited in the graphs below are showing recent increases in the US.

3 Many people are ill (the peak of the epidemic); others have recovered and are immune.

4 A few people are ill; a large number are now immune.

Tuberculosis
The number of cases of tuberculosis is increasing because of growing numbers of people with weakened immune systems as a result of AIDS, malnutrition, or poor hygiene (especially among the homeless), and the arrival of immigrants who are already infected.

Syphilis
The number of cases of syphilis has been increasing steadily in recent years, especially among drug users. The people infected often do not have access to medical care and may engage in high-risk activities such as prostitution or having multiple sex partners.

Measles
The number of cases of measles jumped in 1989. Many children were not being immunized and the vaccine given between 1957 and 1980 was found to be ineffective (see CHILDHOOD IMMUNIZATION PROGRAM *on page 73).*

25

A HISTORICAL VIEW

Infectious diseases, which remain the major cause of death in many parts of the world, have profoundly influenced the course of history. They have been responsible for the redistribution of whole populations and have altered the outcome of wars and even some engineering projects, such as the Panama Canal.

IMPACT OF INFECTIOUS DISEASES

Epidemics of dangerous infectious diseases, such as plague in the 14th century and smallpox in the 17th and 18th centuries, caused sudden decreases in popu-

SPREAD OF PLAGUE

Plague is an infectious disease carried by rodents. It is transmitted to humans by the bites of fleas that have fed on the blood of infected rodents (see below). Epidemics of plague killed millions of people in medieval Europe. Though rare, the disease still exists today in Africa, Asia, and North and South America.

1 The rat flea *Xenopsylla cheopis* (shown below, magnified nine times) lives on a rat and feeds on its blood. If the rat becomes infected with the plague bacterium *Yersinia pestis* and dies, the flea finds a new host. If all the local rats have died of plague, the rat flea resorts to feeding on people.

2 If a flea has taken in blood from an infected rat, its stomach becomes obstructed by plague bacteria. In order to feed again, the flea regurgitates these bacteria, infecting the person in the process.

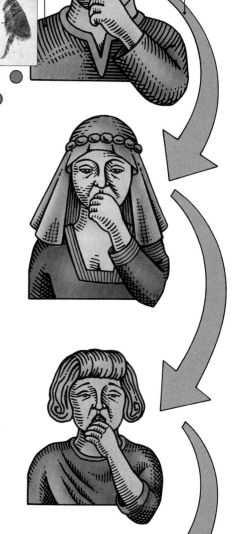

Flea infects person

Spread of infection

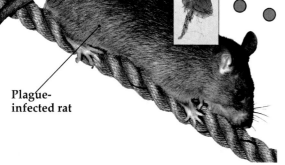

Rat flea

Plague-infected rat

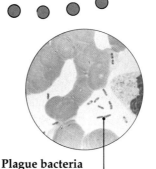

Plague bacteria

Plague in the 14th century
Between 1346 and 1352, a bubonic plague epidemic, spread by the black rat (illustrated below), killed 20 million people throughout Europe.

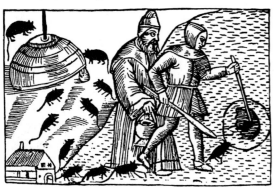

3 Fever develops in infected people. They have chills and a headache and may feel confused and sometimes delirious. The lymph nodes (usually those in the groin) become swollen and pus-filled. These swellings, known as buboes, give the disease its name – bubonic plague. A very severe form of the infection, pneumonic plague, can spread to others by bacteria projected into the air through coughing.

THE FIRST VACCINE

In the mid-18th century, it was discovered that milkmaids who had had cowpox – a disease acquired from infected cows – never contracted smallpox, a more serious disease. The English physician Edward Jenner (1749-1823) tested this phenomenon in experiments (see below). Cowpox vaccination eventually became established as a safe procedure that provided effective immunity against smallpox.

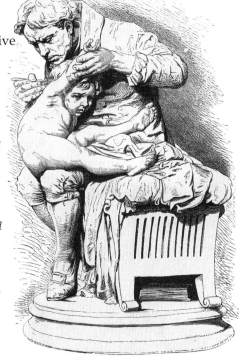

Jenner's cowpox experiment
In 1796, Jenner removed some material from a milkmaid's cowpox pustule and scratched it into the skin of an 8-year-old boy. The mild illness cowpox developed in the boy. Some weeks later, Jenner inoculated the boy, in the same manner, with smallpox. As predicted, the disease failed to develop.

ANTISEPTICS AND STERILE SURGERY

Until the 1860s and Pasteur's germ theory, infection usually followed surgery. English surgeon Joseph Lister (1827-1912) used carbolic acid as an antiseptic. Later, surgical instruments were sterilized by heat. When Hungarian physician Ignaz Semmelweis (1818-1865) urged doctors to wash their hands before delivering babies, deadly infections in women giving birth decreased sharply.

lations in various parts of the world. Devastation occurred when newcomers introduced diseases into previously unaffected populations. For example, in the 16th century, Spanish settlers brought smallpox to the Americas, where the indigenous population had no natural immunity to the disease. During the next century, smallpox killed 90 percent of the native residents.

In most wars before and including World War I, diseases claimed more lives than were lost in battle. The first attempt to dig the Panama Canal was abandoned in 1887 after thousands of workers died of yellow fever and malaria.

Worldwide, infectious diseases continue to be the major cause of death because of their extremely high rates in developing countries. In developed countries, most infections have been brought under control with vaccines, antibiotics, and other advances in medicine, and improvements in living standards and public health.

DISCOVERY OF MICROORGANISMS

In Holland in 1676, Anton van Leeuwenhoek (1632-1723) constructed a powerful single lens microscope that enabled him to observe tiny organisms, or "little animals," as he called them. But it was not until the 19th century that Louis Pasteur (1822-1895) recognized the link between microorganisms and disease (see below).

In 1876, German bacteriologist Robert Koch (1843-1910) proved that a germ is the cause of anthrax (a serious bacterial infection of livestock that is occasionally transmitted to people). Pasteur confirmed this in later experiments and he also proved that rabies was caused by an organism – now known to be a virus – too small to be seen with a microscope. Pasteur developed effective vaccines for both anthrax and rabies.

Pasteur's germ theory of disease
The French chemist Louis Pasteur (below) discovered that fermentation was the result of the activity of microscopic organisms. In 1858, he suggested that human diseases were also caused by specific germs.

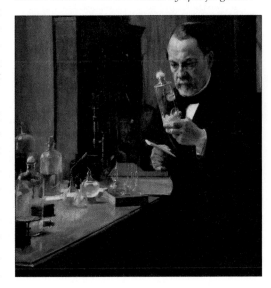

IMPROVEMENTS IN PUBLIC HEALTH

Many doctors at first treated Pasteur's germ theory of disease with contempt. But by the mid-1800s in Europe, even prior to Pasteur's discoveries, the importance of cleanliness and hygienic practices for controlling disease was becoming apparent. Improvements in living standards, personal hygiene, public water supplies, sanitation, and food processing were implemented. As a result, the incidence of many infectious diseases and the number of deaths caused by infections began to decline. This pattern was repeated in other developed countries, including the US (see right and below). Improved medical treatments and the development of antibiotics and effective vaccines also helped reduce the incidence of many infections.

Major causes of death

A hundred years ago, more people in the US died of infections than of any other cause. The number of deaths from infections started to decrease significantly in the 1920s with the development of vaccines for widespread deadly diseases such as diphtheria. The development of antibiotic drugs in the 1930s and 1940s has also helped to control many infectious diseases. The six leading causes of death in 1900 and in 1984 are shown below.

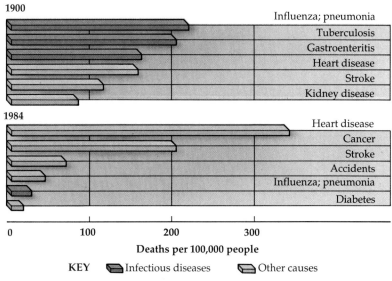

DECLINE OF INFECTIOUS DISEASES

In developed countries, the incidence of many infectious diseases, such as diphtheria, poliomyelitis, scarlet fever, whooping cough, tuberculosis, typhoid fever, and tetanus, has declined dramatically.

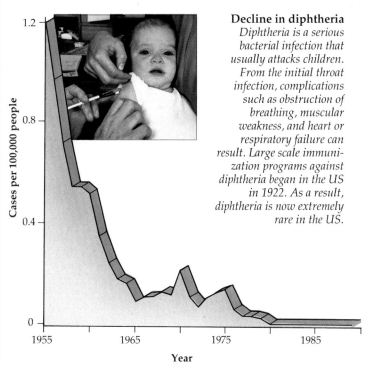

Decline in diphtheria
Diphtheria is a serious bacterial infection that usually attacks children. From the initial throat infection, complications such as obstruction of breathing, muscular weakness, and heart or respiratory failure can result. Large scale immunization programs against diphtheria began in the US in 1922. As a result, diphtheria is now extremely rare in the US.

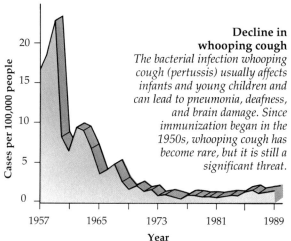

Decline in whooping cough
The bacterial infection whooping cough (pertussis) usually affects infants and young children and can lead to pneumonia, deafness, and brain damage. Since immunization began in the 1950s, whooping cough has become rare, but it is still a significant threat.

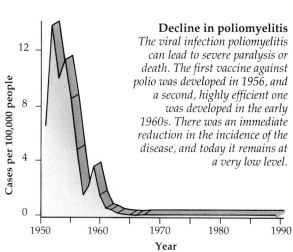

Decline in poliomyelitis
The viral infection poliomyelitis can lead to severe paralysis or death. The first vaccine against polio was developed in 1956, and a second, highly efficient one was developed in the early 1960s. There was an immediate reduction in the incidence of the disease, and today it remains at a very low level.

HOW SMALLPOX HAS BEEN ERADICATED

Smallpox was always one of the most threatening of all infectious diseases. Recurrent epidemics claimed the lives of vast numbers of people and disfigured many survivors. Today, as the result of an intensive global vaccination campaign, smallpox has been completely eradicated throughout the world – a unique success story. The remaining cultures of the viruses, held at the Centers for Disease Control in Atlanta, Georgia, and at the Research Institute for Viral Preparations in Moscow, are scheduled to be destroyed before December 1993.

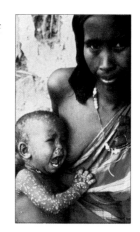

A deadly disease
There were two strains of smallpox virus. Variola major had a death rate of up to 50 percent, while variola minor killed about one in every 100 infected people. The infection caused fever, headache, muscle ache, and nausea. Pus-filled blisters (shown left) that covered the face, arms, and chest of victims left disfiguring scars.

A worldwide vaccination program
In 1967, the World Health Organization began an intensive, international vaccination program to eliminate smallpox. The map below shows the regions where the disease was still present in 1967, 1972, and 1975. The last reported case of smallpox, in October 1977, was a 23 year old from Somalia. In October 1979, the World Health Organization officially declared the world smallpox-free.

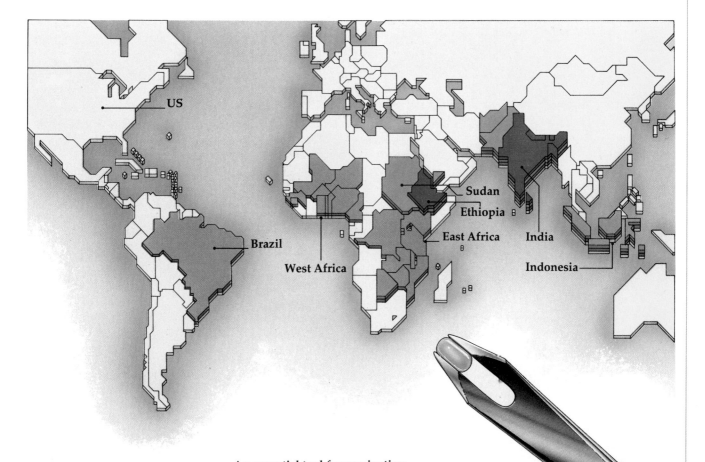

US

Sudan
Ethiopia
Brazil
West Africa
East Africa
India
Indonesia

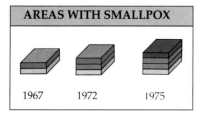

AREAS WITH SMALLPOX		
1967	1972	1975

An essential tool for vaccination
In remote parts of the world with primitive facilities, a simple vaccination technique was vital. The forked (bifurcated) needle (shown here greatly enlarged) fulfilled the need. When dipped into the vaccine, the needle held one drop between its prongs, sufficient for one vaccination. The needle was held perpendicular to the skin and 15 rapid punctures were made just beneath the skin within the smallest area possible – about ⅛ inch in diameter. With this method, only a tiny amount of vaccine was needed per person.

CURRENT PERSPECTIVES

The incidence of several infectious diseases is closely monitored by a branch of the federal government called the Centers for Disease Control (CDC), which is the primary force for disease prevention in the US. Each week, state health departments notify the CDC of the number of cases of these designated illnesses that have been reported in their state.

Reportable infections are those with the potential to cause epidemics (widespread illness throughout a population). The 20 reportable infections that occurred most frequently in 1989 are charted on page 31. Public health measures to identify the people at risk and institute treatment and prevention programs can be effective in controlling these particular illnesses. Many other common infections, such as influenza, are not reportable, however. The CDC has established a surveillance system to determine if an influenza virus is causing a large number of deaths or if a new strain of the virus is causing epidemics. The validity of this monitoring system depends on the accuracy of death certificates.

Newspaper headlines
Media coverage of infectious diseases – particularly sexually transmitted diseases and "new" diseases such as Lyme disease – has increased in recent years. Such coverage can play a useful role in educating the public on the importance of vaccinating children, following safe sex procedures, and modifying life-style to avoid disease.

Centers for Disease Control
The Centers for Disease Control (CDC) tracks infectious diseases, solves medical mysteries, and helps prevent disease throughout the world. Since it was founded in 1946, the agency has launched intensive immunization programs that have dramatically reduced the incidence of the most serious infectious childhood diseases. In 1981, the CDC reported the first five cases of the new disease AIDS.

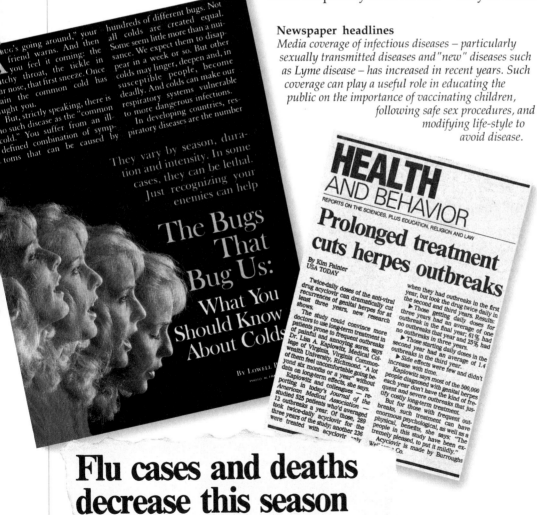

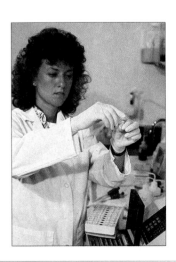

GROUPS OF INFECTIONS

Sexually transmitted diseases

Sexually transmitted diseases continue to be an increasingly serious health problem in the US. Gonorrhea, syphilis, and acquired immune deficiency syndrome (AIDS) are among the top six most common reportable diseases. Viral infections – such as genital warts and herpes – and infections with chlamydia (a type of bacteria) have occurred at a startlingly high rate over the past 20 years (see SEXUALLY TRANSMITTED DISEASES on page 130).

Childhood infections

Successful immunization programs have made measles, mumps, rubella, and whooping cough (pertussis) rare in the US today. Recently, however, an increase in measles cases (among teenagers who were immunized with an ineffective vaccine and among unvaccinated children) has led to a recommendation for a follow-up measles vaccination (see CHILDHOOD INFECTIONS on page 88).

Viral hepatitis

Hepatitis is caused by many different viruses (see VIRAL HEPATITIS on page 116). The hepatitis B and C viruses can be transmitted by unsterile needles, infected blood or blood products, or during sexual intercourse. Health care workers and other people who are at risk should be vaccinated against hepatitis B.

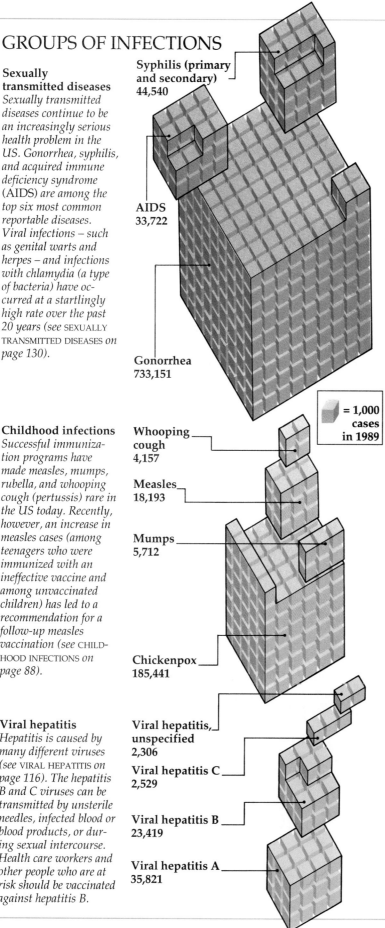

Syphilis (primary and secondary)
44,540

AIDS
33,722

Gonorrhea
733,151

= 1,000 cases in 1989

Whooping cough
4,157

Measles
18,193

Mumps
5,712

Chickenpox
185,441

Viral hepatitis, unspecified
2,306

Viral hepatitis C
2,529

Viral hepatitis B
23,419

Viral hepatitis A
35,821

Gastrointestinal infections

Many gastrointestinal infections caused by viruses are relatively mild. But bacteria are a common cause of gastroenteritis, a severe diarrheal illness. Salmonella bacteria are a frequent source of food poisoning. Because of debilitating effects, including dehydration from diarrhea and vomiting, these infections can be fatal (see DIGESTIVE TRACT INFECTIONS on page 110).

Salmonellosis (excluding typhoid fever)
47,812

Shigellosis
25,010

Amebiasis
3,217

Lung infections

Bronchitis and pneumonia (see LUNG INFECTIONS on page 102) are more likely to affect smokers and people with weakened immune systems. But legionnaires' disease – a type of pneumonia – kills a few healthy, young to middle-aged adults each year. By the 1970s, tuberculosis had declined in the US, but it is now reappearing in some groups, such as people with AIDS, migrant farm workers, and the homeless.

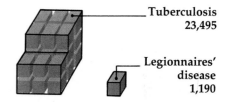

Tuberculosis
23,495

Legionnaires' disease
1,190

Brain infections

Meningitis, an infection of the membranes that cover the brain, can be caused by viruses or bacteria. Bacterial meningitis is very serious; it causes brain damage or death in about 28 percent of cases. Encephalitis, an infection of the brain itself, is usually caused by a virus. It is less common than meningitis, but can be serious (see BRAIN INFECTIONS on page 92).

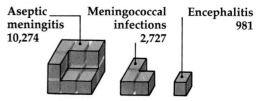

Aseptic meningitis
10,274

Meningococcal infections
2,727

Encephalitis
981

Malaria

Between 1,000 and 2,000 cases of malaria are diagnosed in the US each year. Most cases occur in immigrants from Southeast Asia or in Americans who visit areas where the disease is present.

Malaria
1,277

HOSPITAL-ACQUIRED INFECTIONS

About 5 to 6 percent of patients acquire an infection while in the hospital. These infections occur as a result of exposure to germs and weakened resistance to infections. Some hospital infections are inevitable. Many people admitted to hospitals have progressive, incurable diseases that make them vulnerable to

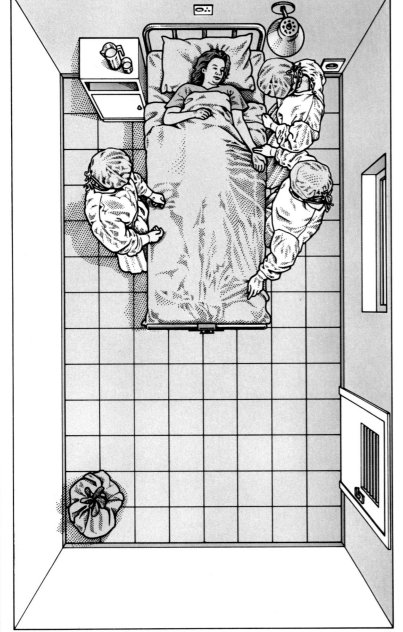

illnesses such as pneumonia and urinary tract infections. Treatments such as organ transplantation and chemotherapy for cancer include the use of drugs that suppress the body's immune defense system. Surgery carries a small but unavoidable risk of infection at the site of the incision. Many hospital infections are caused by bacteria that have become resistant to antibiotics, making these illnesses more difficult to treat.

Preventing hospital infections

Most researchers agree that a substantial percentage of hospital infections could be prevented. All American hospitals have infection control programs that include monitoring patients and hospital staff for infections, and studying disease organisms in the laboratory to determine whether they are becoming resistant to certain antibiotics.

This continuing surveillance identifies hospital wards or units in which the infection rate has increased. Ideally, such monitoring reveals the cause of an outbreak and makes early intervention possible. For instance, a sudden rise in the number of infections among patients with urinary catheters would trigger an investigation into whether the sterilization procedures used to prepare the catheters were adequate and whether staff members were following proper procedures. The rate of infection following surgery is much lower today than 10 or 20 years ago as a result of antibiotics and improved surgical techniques and sterilization procedures.

Isolation
Hospitalized patients with highly contagious or dangerous infections may need to be isolated to prevent the spread of disease organisms to staff, visitors, and other patients. Precautionary procedures vary according to the infection. For some respiratory infections, such as pneumonia that is caused by antibiotic-resistant bacteria, visitors and staff should wear masks. For patients with infected wounds or gastrointestinal infections, visitors may need to wear gowns and gloves.

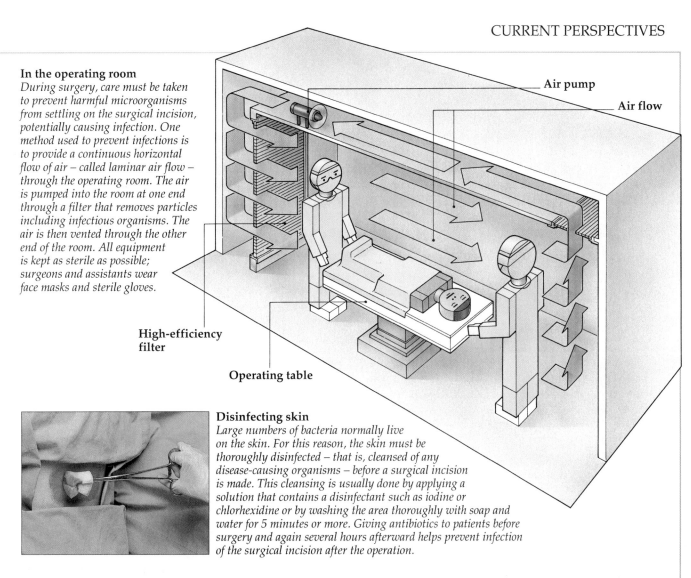

In the operating room
During surgery, care must be taken to prevent harmful microorganisms from settling on the surgical incision, potentially causing infection. One method used to prevent infections is to provide a continuous horizontal flow of air – called laminar air flow – through the operating room. The air is pumped into the room at one end through a filter that removes particles including infectious organisms. The air is then vented through the other end of the room. All equipment is kept as sterile as possible; surgeons and assistants wear face masks and sterile gloves.

Air pump

Air flow

High-efficiency filter

Operating table

Disinfecting skin
Large numbers of bacteria normally live on the skin. For this reason, the skin must be thoroughly disinfected – that is, cleansed of any disease-causing organisms – before a surgical incision is made. This cleansing is usually done by applying a solution that contains a disinfectant such as iodine or chlorhexidine or by washing the area thoroughly with soap and water for 5 minutes or more. Giving antibiotics to patients before surgery and again several hours afterward helps prevent infection of the surgical incision after the operation.

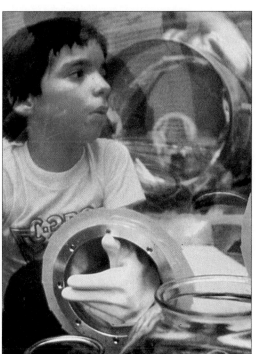

Protective isolation
Some hospitalized patients need protection from germs because their immune systems are weakened. In such cases, all visitors and staff must wear gowns, masks, and gloves to protect the patient. In rare cases of severe suppression of the immune system, the patient lives in a specially constructed sterile room, or "bubble," as shown at left, into which only filtered air can enter.

Autoclave
Surgical instruments and other hospital equipment are sterilized in an apparatus called an autoclave. The autoclave kills microorganisms by producing steam under very high pressure. A gauge automatically regulates the pressure and degree of heat inside the sealed chamber.

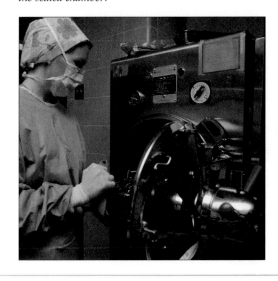

RESISTANCE TO DRUGS

The ability of some microorganisms to develop resistance to drugs used against them is a persistent problem in the fight against infectious diseases.

Developing resistance

Bacteria, fungi, and other microorganisms live in a highly competitive world. When their environment changes, creating a threat to their existence, some organisms are able to survive because they have inherited specific properties that enable them to neutralize the new threat. The life span of a bacterium is measured in minutes or hours. Therefore, if an antibiotic wipes out 99 percent of a bacterial population, within a couple of days a new population of bacteria will emerge. These bacteria, which are all descendants of the 1 percent of survivors, will possess the trait that makes them resistant to the new threat.

The way in which bacteria develop resistance to antibiotics over a period of time is shown in the box below.

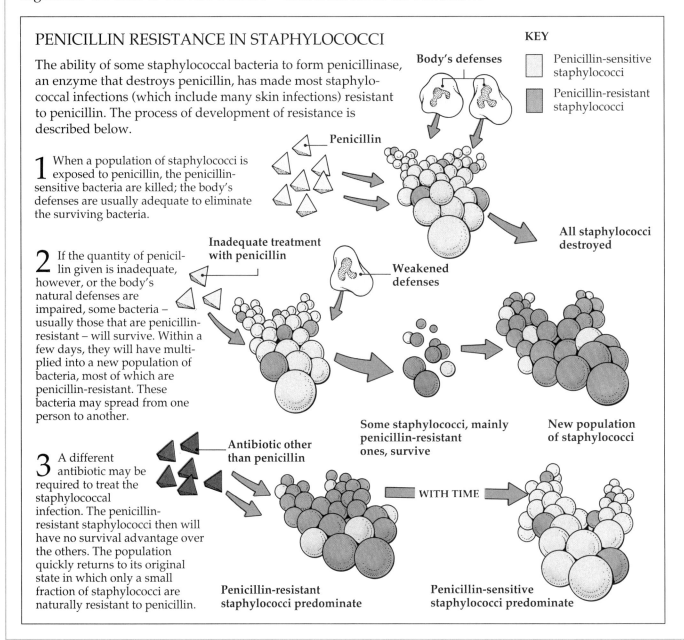

PENICILLIN RESISTANCE IN STAPHYLOCOCCI

KEY
☐ Penicillin-sensitive staphylococci
■ Penicillin-resistant staphylococci

The ability of some staphylococcal bacteria to form penicillinase, an enzyme that destroys penicillin, has made most staphylococcal infections (which include many skin infections) resistant to penicillin. The process of development of resistance is described below.

1 When a population of staphylococci is exposed to penicillin, the penicillin-sensitive bacteria are killed; the body's defenses are usually adequate to eliminate the surviving bacteria.

Body's defenses

Penicillin

All staphylococci destroyed

2 If the quantity of penicillin given is inadequate, however, or the body's natural defenses are impaired, some bacteria – usually those that are penicillin-resistant – will survive. Within a few days, they will have multiplied into a new population of bacteria, most of which are penicillin-resistant. These bacteria may spread from one person to another.

Inadequate treatment with penicillin

Weakened defenses

Some staphylococci, mainly penicillin-resistant ones, survive

New population of staphylococci

3 A different antibiotic may be required to treat the staphylococcal infection. The penicillin-resistant staphylococci then will have no survival advantage over the others. The population quickly returns to its original state in which only a small fraction of staphylococci are naturally resistant to penicillin.

Antibiotic other than penicillin

WITH TIME

Penicillin-resistant staphylococci predominate

Penicillin-sensitive staphylococci predominate

Plasmids and resistance

Bacteria have been exposed to antibiotics for 50 years now. This has been enough time for many of these organisms to develop elaborate mechanisms of resistance to bacteria-fighting drugs.

The most powerful defense mechanism is the ability of some bacteria to transfer resistance among themselves. They do this by sharing tiny packages of DNA called plasmids, which contain inherited material – in this case, the resistant genes (see TRANSFER OF RESISTANCE at right). As a result of this type of genetic transfer, many populations of bacteria today are able to make enzymes called beta-lactamases. These enzymes provide bacteria with the ability to neutralize the effects of many different types of antibiotics. Super-resistant strains of bacteria that have the ability to protect themselves against several classes of antibiotics also have evolved. In a similar way, some protozoa have developed resistance to drugs used against them. For example, in many parts of the world, malaria parasites have become resistant to some of the antimalarial drugs used for both prevention and cure.

Discouraging resistance

Three main approaches are used to help prevent the development of antibiotic-resistant bacteria.

First, doctors are careful in prescribing antibiotics today. The more widely antibiotics are used, the more likely it is that antibiotic-resistant strains of bacteria will emerge. Second, it is important that patients take the full prescribed course of an antibiotic to ensure that all the disease-causing bacteria are destroyed. Third, modern pharmacology has provided a wide spectrum of antibiotics from which doctors can choose. This enables them to prescribe the antibiotic that is most specific for a particular infection, thereby reducing the risk that a person's normal bacteria will develop resistance while he or she is taking the drug.

TRANSFER OF RESISTANCE

Plasmids are tiny packages of hereditary information (DNA) that can transfer antibiotic resistance very rapidly through a population of bacteria.

1 Some bacteria have plasmids that contain genetic coding for the production of antibiotic-resistant substances.

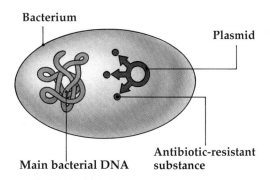

Bacterium

Plasmid

Main bacterial DNA

Antibiotic-resistant substance

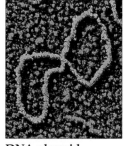

DNA plasmid
The color-enhanced photograph above shows a plasmid of bacterial DNA (magnified 140,000 times). In addition to genes that provide antibiotic resistance, plasmids may contain genes that confer other characteristics, such as an increased ability to cause disease.

2 Plasmids can be transferred among bacteria by a process called conjugation. First, the plasmid duplicates itself inside the "donor" bacterium. A microscopic, tube-like structure, called a pilus, on the surface of the donor bacterium is then inserted into a recipient bacterium. The plasmid then passes into the recipient via this tiny tube. The photograph at left (magnified 7,400 times) shows conjugating bacteria.

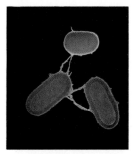

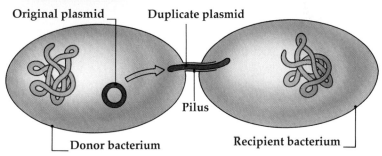

Original plasmid

Duplicate plasmid

Pilus

Donor bacterium

Recipient bacterium

3 Both donor and recipient bacteria are now able to make the substance that provides antibiotic resistance.

Antibiotic-resistant substance

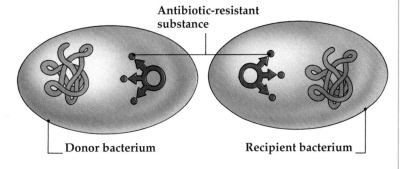

Donor bacterium

Recipient bacterium

CHAPTER TWO

DISEASE ORGANISMS

MICROORGANISMS were first discovered in the 17th century after the invention of the microscope, but more than 200 years passed before Louis Pasteur proved that microbes caused infections in people. In 1880, German bacteriologist Robert Koch established a set of guidelines for determining that a specific microorganism causes a specific disease. These rules, known as Koch's postulates, are as follows: the microorganism must be found in every person or animal that has the disease; the microorganism must be isolated in the laboratory; and isolated microorganisms must reproduce the disease in animals and be recovered from their infected tissues. Koch's rules established the field of medical microbiology as a science. Less than 20 years after the guidelines were established, Koch and his pupils had identified many of the most common disease-causing bacteria as well as the illnesses they produced. However, the research team was unable to link microorganisms to a number of diseases that were obviously infectious. Fluid extracts from infected tissues were still infectious after being passed through filters that removed bacteria. The organisms therefore had to be smaller than bacteria. They were named "filterable viruses." Later

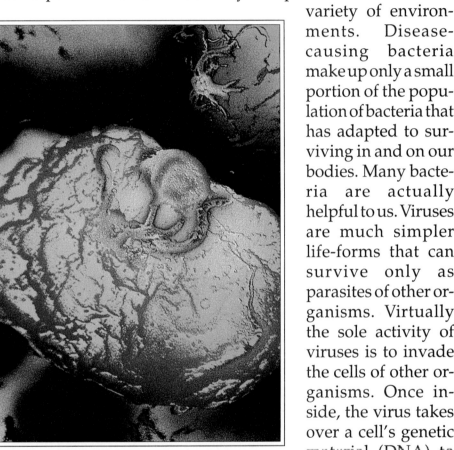

they became known simply as viruses. Bacteria and viruses are responsible for a significant number of infections that occur today. These two large groups of microorganisms – highlighted in this chapter – are very different. Bacteria are among the oldest forms of life. They are neither plant nor animal, but are instead in a biological category of their own. Bacteria are capable of a relatively independent existence in a variety of environments. Disease-causing bacteria make up only a small portion of the population of bacteria that has adapted to surviving in and on our bodies. Many bacteria are actually helpful to us. Viruses are much simpler life-forms that can survive only as parasites of other organisms. Virtually the sole activity of viruses is to invade the cells of other organisms. Once inside, the virus takes over a cell's genetic material (DNA) to make copies of itself and cause disease.

Along with bacteria and viruses, two other groups of organisms are a significant source of infections. Fungi (which include yeasts and molds) can cause some less dangerous but troublesome infections, often confined to the skin and mucous membranes. Animal parasites include both single-celled animals such as protozoa and multicelled organisms such as worms.

BACTERIA

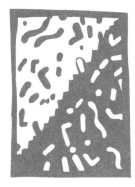

BACTERIA ARE TINY ORGANISMS that inhabit the world around us. They live in the air, soil, and water; on our furniture and clothes; and in and on our bodies. Most bacteria are harmless and, in fact, perform beneficial functions. Many of the bacteria in our bodies protect us against the harmful effects of other organisms. But when they enter internal tissues, bacteria can cause disease.

Bacteria are the smallest free-living organisms – that is, they support their own growth and reproduction. These microscopic organisms are only about one thousandth of a millimeter in size. Their shapes vary. Cocci, which are spherical, and bacilli, which are rod-shaped, are two of the most common types. Less frequently, bacteria are shaped like commas, kidneys, or spirals. Individual species tend to cluster to-gether in particular patterns, such as chains, pyramids, or clumps.

STRUCTURE OF A BACTERIUM

Each bacterium is a single-celled organism. Unlike animal cells – which exist as individual units of a highly organized system such as the human body – a bacterium is able to survive on its own. Its structure provides it with protection and the ability to acquire nutrients, move, reproduce, and attach itself to surfaces where it can thrive.

Ribosome
Ribosomes, found inside the cell, are the sites where proteins are formed. Bacteria require proteins to grow and reproduce.

Nucleoid region

How bacteria reproduce
A bacterium increases in size and divides in two after a new cell wall forms across the middle. The process can repeat itself rapidly. From a single bacterium, 1 million bacteria can develop within 10 hours if sufficient nutrients are available.

Bacterial chromosome
The genetic (inherited) material of the bacterium is usually contained inside a single chromosome, composed of one large, circular molecule of DNA. The chromosome exists in the cytoplasm; the area occupied by the DNA is called the nucleoid region. Some bacteria also contain tiny packages of genetic material called plasmids.

Slime layer
In addition to a cell wall, a bacterium may be coated with a slime layer, which prevents the organism from dehydrating and losing nutrients. The slime layer also enables it to attach to surfaces or other bacteria.

Plasma membrane (or cytoplasmic membrane)
The plasma membrane, located inside the cell wall, is the inner boundary layer of the cell. It regulates the entry and exit of chem-ical substances necessary for cell function.

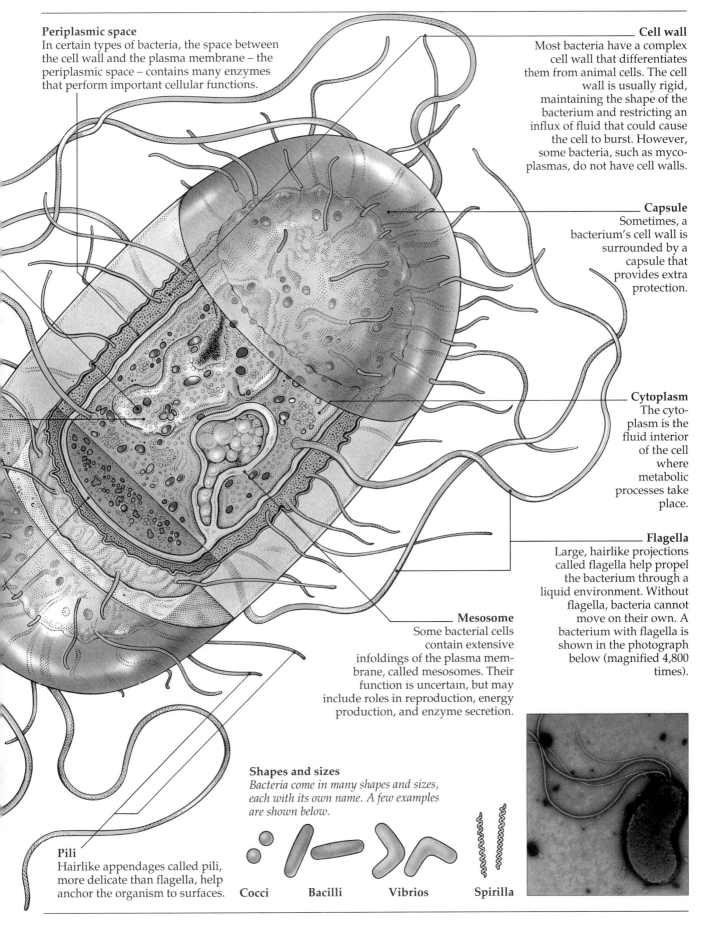

Periplasmic space
In certain types of bacteria, the space between the cell wall and the plasma membrane – the periplasmic space – contains many enzymes that perform important cellular functions.

Cell wall
Most bacteria have a complex cell wall that differentiates them from animal cells. The cell wall is usually rigid, maintaining the shape of the bacterium and restricting an influx of fluid that could cause the cell to burst. However, some bacteria, such as mycoplasmas, do not have cell walls.

Capsule
Sometimes, a bacterium's cell wall is surrounded by a capsule that provides extra protection.

Cytoplasm
The cytoplasm is the fluid interior of the cell where metabolic processes take place.

Flagella
Large, hairlike projections called flagella help propel the bacterium through a liquid environment. Without flagella, bacteria cannot move on their own. A bacterium with flagella is shown in the photograph below (magnified 4,800 times).

Mesosome
Some bacterial cells contain extensive infoldings of the plasma membrane, called mesosomes. Their function is uncertain, but may include roles in reproduction, energy production, and enzyme secretion.

Shapes and sizes
Bacteria come in many shapes and sizes, each with its own name. A few examples are shown below.

Cocci **Bacilli** **Vibrios** **Spirilla**

Pili
Hairlike appendages called pili, more delicate than flagella, help anchor the organism to surfaces.

TYPES OF BACTERIA

Most pathogenic bacteria – those that cause disease – can be divided into two main groups according to their reaction to a test called Gram's stain. This test is an important tool to help doctors choose the best antibiotic to treat a specific type of bacterial infection before other laboratory results are available (see DIAGNOSING INFECTIOUS DISEASES on page 76). Depending on their staining properties, bacteria are classified as either gram-positive or gram-negative. Some bacteria – such as chlamydiae, rickettsiae (see UNUSUAL BACTERIA on page 42), and spirochetes – cannot be classified according to the Gram's stain.

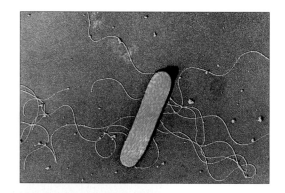

Clostridia

Clostridia live harmlessly in the intestines of people and animals and in soil, but some types can infect wounds or cause illness. Clostridium perfringens *(shown in the photograph below, magnified 600 times)* causes gas gangrene (tissue death). Clostridium difficile *can cause antibiotic-induced diarrhea.*

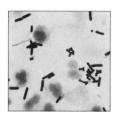

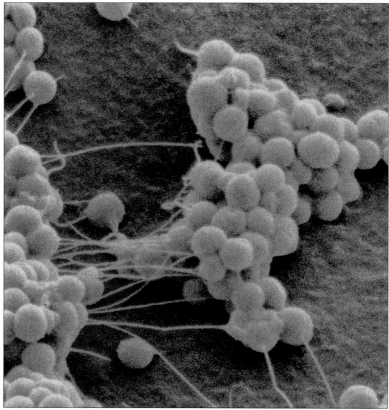

Listeria

If Listeria monocytogenes *(shown in the color-enhanced photograph above, magnified 10,000 times) infects a pregnant woman, the fetus or newborn may be affected.* Listeria *infections have occurred after people have eaten contaminated cheeses and cold, cooked meats.*

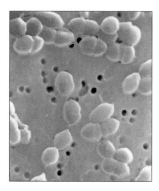

Streptococci

Streptococci tend to form chains, as shown in the color-enhanced photograph above (magnified 5,000 times). Streptococcus pyogenes *causes strep throat and many other infections;* Streptococcus pneumoniae *is a major cause of pneumonia and meningitis.*

Staphylococci

Staphylococci can cause skin infections, such as boils, pustules, and abscesses, and infections in bones, joints, and wounds. Staphylococcus epidermidis *(shown in the color-enhanced photograph above, magnified 33,000 times) normally lives harmlessly on the skin. However, if it enters artificial joints or heart valves during surgery, it can produce dangerous infections.*

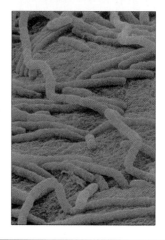

Bacilli

Bacilli are found in soil and water and are carried by animals and insects. Bacillus cereus *(shown in the photograph at left, magnified 2,400 times) can cause food poisoning.* Bacillus anthracis *causes anthrax, which can produce open sores on the skin.*

▲ Pseudomonads

Pseudomonads can occur harmlessly in the gastrointestinal tract but may cause disease in people whose immune systems are impaired. Pseudomonas aeruginosa, *shown in the color-enhanced photograph below (magnified 17,000 times), causes pneumonia, and wound or urinary tract infections.*

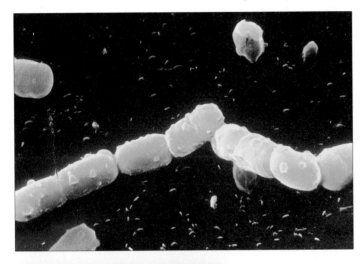

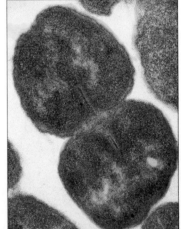

▲ Coliforms

Coliforms are a group of intestinal organisms. Many coliforms live harmlessly in the gastrointestinal systems of people and animals. However, they sometimes cause urinary tract infections or gastroenteritis, a severe diarrheal illness. Salmonella enteritidis, *the organism shown in the color-enhanced photograph above (magnified 6,500 times), can cause acute gastroenteritis.*

▲ Neisseriae

Neisseria *organisms are responsible for several serious infections.* Neisseria gonorrhoeae, *shown in the color-enhanced photograph at left (magnified 39,000 times), causes the sexually transmitted disease gonorrhea.* Neisseria meningitidis *is a major source of meningitis in older children and young adults.*

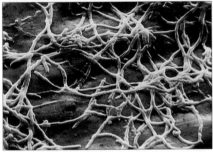

▲ Legionellae

There are several species of legionella bacteria. Legionella pneumophila, *shown in the color-enhanced photograph above (magnified 5,000 times), causes legionnaires' disease, an often life-threatening form of pneumonia.*

● Spirochetes

Spirochetes are spiral-shaped bacteria that are resistant to laboratory staining and therefore cannot be classified as gram-negative or gram-positive. Spirochetes include the organisms responsible for syphilis and leptospirosis (an uncommon disease transmitted to people indirectly from rodents or domestic animals such as dogs). The species of leptospira *shown in the color-enhanced photograph at right (magnified 60,000 times) shows the characteristic spiral formation.*

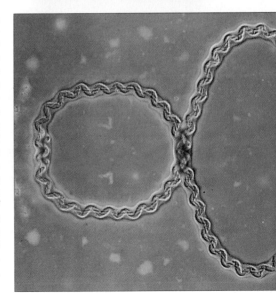

KEY

■ Gram-positive bacteria

▲ Gram-negative bacteria

● Unclassifiable bacteria

OTHER SIGNIFICANT ORGANISMS

Campylobacter organisms are comma-shaped bacteria that are the source of a number of diarrheal illnesses transmitted by animals (see DISEASES ACQUIRED FROM ANIMALS on page 16). Bacteroides, which live in the colon, are anaerobic – that is, they can live without oxygen. These bacteria may spread during colon surgery and cause infections. Mycobacteria are slow-growing bacteria that are resistant to the body's defenses. One species of mycobacteria, which causes tuberculosis, can remain dormant in the body after the primary infection, but may be reactivated. Another mycobacterium is responsible for leprosy. Mycoplasmas resemble bacteria but have no cell walls. They cause infections primarily in the respiratory and genital tracts.

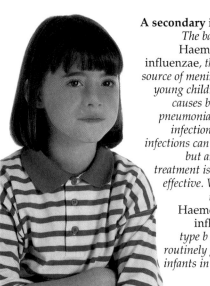

A secondary invader
The bacterium Haemophilus influenzae, *the major source of meningitis in young children, also causes bronchial pneumonia and ear infections. These infections can be fatal, but antibiotic treatment is usually effective. Vaccinations for* Haemophilus influenzae *type b are now routinely given to infants in the US.*

BACTERIA AND DISEASE

Hundreds of types of bacteria are found in the environment and in animals, but relatively few are pathogenic – that is, able to cause disease.

Symptoms occur when your immune system mounts a counterattack against invading organisms. Symptoms of illness

UNUSUAL BACTERIA

Two important groups of disease-causing organisms are chlamydiae and rickettsiae. They are small bacteria, but, like viruses, they can reproduce only by entering a host cell and utilizing its metabolic processes.

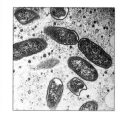

Rickettsiae
Rickettsia rickettsii, *shown in the cells of a tick in the color-enhanced photograph at left (magnified 9,000 times), causes Rocky Mountain spotted fever. Other rickettsiae cause typhus and a type of pneumonia. Some rickettsial infections develop after contact with tick-infested animals; others are spread by infected body lice.*

Chlamydiae
Chlamydia trachomatis *causes eye and genitourinary infections in humans.* Chlamydia psittaci *(shown in the color-enhanced photograph at right, magnified 42,000 times) can be transmitted from birds to people by contact with dust from bird feathers or droppings, causing psittacosis, a pneumonialike infection.* Chlamydia pneumoniae *has recently been found to be a cause of a type of pneumonia.*

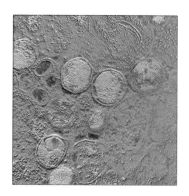

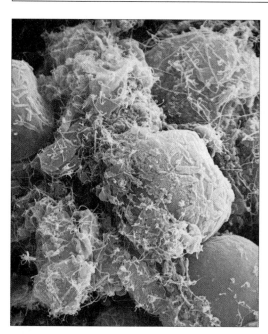

Friendly bacteria
A number of harmless bacteria live in our gastrointestinal tracts and are known as the normal flora (cobweblike structures shown above on intestinal cells, magnified 3,000 times). They help protect us from unfriendly, harmful organisms. But when these helpful bacteria are destroyed, usually by antibiotics, the body becomes vulnerable to disease-causing organisms (pathogens).

SURVIVAL OF BACTERIA

Dryness and excessive heat inhibit bacterial growth. A temperature of 162°F, which is used to pasteurize milk, kills many bacteria; few bacteria survive boiling at 212°F for 10 minutes. Some bacteria form into spores, which can withstand greater extremes of temperature and lack of water and nutrients. For this reason, hospital equipment, including surgical instruments, are sterilized through a combination of steam, heat, and pressure in a machine called an autoclave (see page 33).

are also produced by two different kinds of toxins that the organisms make. Endotoxins, small parts of the bacterial cell wall, can cause fever and shock. Exotoxins, which are excreted by the bacteria, can cause symptoms such as diarrhea. To produce symptoms, pathogens must be strong enough to overcome your body's defenses (see THE BODY'S DEFENSES on page 62).

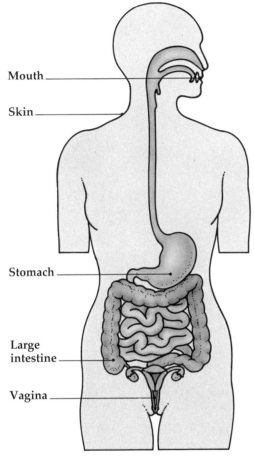

Location of resident bacteria
Most of the bacteria that normally inhabit the body live in the large intestine; they include Bacteroides, Escherichia, *and* Enterobacter *organisms. Bacteria also colonize the skin, mouth, and vagina. Very few can live in the stomach because of its acidic environment.*

Mouth

Skin

Stomach

Large intestine

Vagina

ANTIBIOTIC DRUGS

Antibiotics are drugs used to treat infections caused by bacteria. Originally derived from living organisms, many antibiotic drugs are now made synthetically.

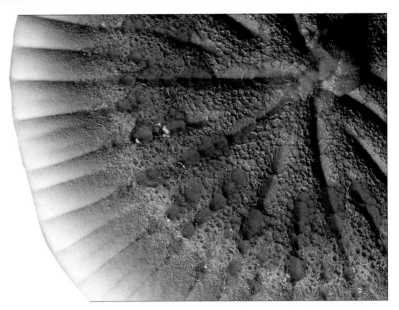

Valuable extract from a fungus
In 1929, Alexander Fleming noted that bacterial colonies growing on a culture plate were destroyed after they were contaminated by a mold, Penicillium notatum *(shown above). In 1940, scientists at Oxford University in England isolated and purified penicillin, the antibiotic secreted by the mold, and first used it to treat a man with a severe lung infection.*

Penicillin, derived from a fungus (see above), was the first antibiotic to be discovered. Its first large-scale use was as a treatment for wounds suffered by troops during World War II. More antibiotics – tetracyclines, erythromycin, streptomycin and other aminoglycosides were developed after the war.

In the mid 1950s, pharmaceutical industry scientists produced variations of penicillin that were effective against a wider range of disease-causing bacteria. But some bacteria are able to produce enzymes – beta-lactamases – that block the effectiveness of penicillin. To fight these penicillin-destroying enzymes, antibiotics such as vancomycin and cephalosporins were developed.

Quinolones, the newest class of synthetically made antibiotics, are effective against many types of bacteria, including coliforms (see page 41). In recent years, strains of bacteria – notably staphylococci – have emerged that are resistant to drugs that were previously effective against them. The search continues for new antibiotics, as well as effective new combinations and variations.

ADVERSE EFFECTS OF DRUGS

Interference with liver or kidney function, damage to growing bones or cartilage, and toxic or allergic reactions are possible side effects of taking antibiotics. Adverse reactions may also occur if the dose is too high or if the antibiotic interacts with other drugs. A drug prescribed to treat a specific infection sometimes acts against the body's normal bacteria, such as those that inhabit the gastrointestinal tract. These areas may then become prone to invasion by other disease-causing organisms. Many yeast infections develop in this way.

Antibiotics in liquid form
Most antibiotics are available as liquids, which are useful for children or people with sore throats.

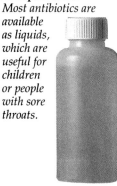

Methods of administration

Antibiotics are usually taken as tablets, capsules, or liquids. The drugs are absorbed from the gastrointestinal tract into the bloodstream and then carried in the blood to the site of infection. Three or four doses a day are usually required. However, newer antibiotics that are taken only once or twice a day have recently become available.

In people who are more seriously ill, antibiotics may be given by direct injec-tion or gradual infusion into a vein. In this way, the full dose of the drug reaches the bloodstream much more quickly than if the drug were taken by mouth. Antibiotics are sometimes injected into muscle tissue, providing a rapid but often brief effect. A few antibiotics that are not absorbed by the gastrointestinal system can be given only by injection. Antibiotics may also be applied directly to the skin, eyes, or vagina in the form of ointments, drops, or suppositories.

HOW DRUGS COMBAT BACTERIA

Bacteriostatic and bactericidal are terms used to describe how antibiotics disable bacteria. The effects that different drugs have on specific parts of a bacterium are shown below.

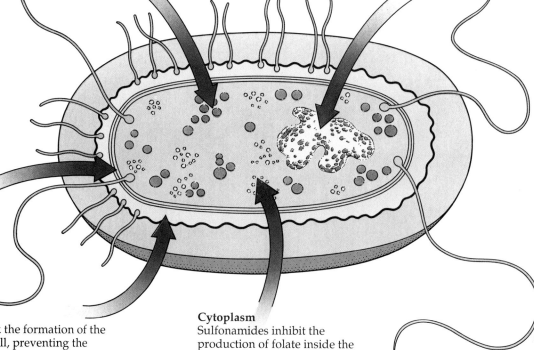

Bacteriostatic agents
These drugs do not destroy bacteria; they make them incapable of reproducing, thereby limiting the harm they can cause. Drugs with a bacteriostatic action work by damaging the bacterium's plasma membrane or by inhibiting one or more stages in the cell's growth or replication.

Ribosomes
Chloramphenicol, tetracyclines, and erythromycin inhibit protein production by structures called ribosomes inside the bacterium.

Bactericidal agents
These drugs kill bacteria. Some bactericidal agents work by destroying the organism's cell wall, causing its contents to leak out. Other bactericidal drugs prevent the bacteria from making essential proteins. In some cases, a drug that is bactericidal (lethal to bacteria) at high doses may be bacteriostatic (damaging to bacteria) at lower doses. Bactericidal drugs are used to treat serious infections.

Genetic material
A group of drugs that includes rifampin, which is used to treat tuberculosis, blocks RNA production. The lack of RNA prevents the bacterium from making vital proteins. The quinolones block the action of an enzyme necessary for bacterial reproduction.

Plasma membrane
A group of drugs called polymyx-ins disrupts the structure of the plasma mem-brane.

Cell wall
Penicillins block the formation of the bacterial cell wall, preventing the organism from reproducing and eventually causing its destruction.

Cytoplasm
Sulfonamides inhibit the production of folate inside the bacterium's cytoplasm. Folate is an important vitamin.

MAIN TYPES OF ANTIBIOTICS

Penicillin and penicillin-type antibiotics

Penicillin is effective against some streptococci; ampicillin and amoxicillin are effective against streptococci and some coliforms. Some penicillin-type antibiotics that are susceptible to beta-lactamase (an antibiotic-destroying substance produced by some bacteria) can be mixed with beta-lactamase blockers to extend the range of bacteria they can destroy. Drugs that are not vulnerable to beta-lactamase have also been developed. These antibiotics have few side effects because they act only against bacterial cell walls.

Cephalosporins

Cephalosporins act in a similar way to penicillin, but have a slightly different structure that makes them more resistant to beta-lactamase, the antibiotic-destroying substance. These antibiotics are active against streptococci, staphylococci, and coliforms, and are often given before surgery to prevent infections from occurring after the operation. Imipenem is a cephalosporinlike agent that kills many types of bacteria.

Monobactams

Monobactams are structurally similar to other beta-lactamase-resistant antibiotics. They are active only against certain bacteria and are often taken by people who have allergies to penicillin.

Erythromycin

Erythromycin is effective against most streptococci and staphylococci, mycoplasmas, chlamydiae, and *Campylobacter* organisms; it is also useful in treating legionnaires' disease. Nausea is a common side effect.

Carbapenems

Carbapenems have a unique structure that conveys resistance to antibiotic-destroying substances, making the drugs effective against many types of bacteria. One disadvantage of these antibiotics is that resistant bacteria or fungi may develop in the body while the person is taking the drug.

Tetracyclines

These antibiotics are effective against mycoplasmas, chlamydiae, rickettsiae, and some streptococci. They are not used to treat children or pregnant women because they are incorporated into growing teeth and bone.

Clindamycin

Clindamycin is used to treat staphylococcal infections and infections caused by anaerobic bacteria, which do not require oxygen to live.

Aminoglycosides

Aminoglycosides are used to treat blood poisoning, abdominal infections, and infections in people who are particularly susceptible to bacterial invasion, such as cancer patients. However, because these antibiotics can cause hearing loss, loss of balance, and kidney problems, the amount of the drug circulating in the blood must be carefully monitored.

Synthetic antibiotics

Quinolones are derivatives of an older synthetically produced drug, nalidixic acid. They are active against streptococci, staphylococci, coliforms, and pseudomonads. Quinolones are not used to treat children or pregnant women because they can interfere with the growth of cartilage. Trimethoprim is used to treat urinary tract infections and some types of gastroenteritis. The first synthetic antibiotics, the sulfonamides, were used in the 1930s, before penicillin was developed. Today, sulfonamides are usually used along with other agents.

Metronidazole

Metronidazole is effective in treating infections caused by anaerobic bacteria, which live without oxygen, and some parasites.

ASK YOUR DOCTOR ANTIBIOTICS

Q **The symptoms from my strep throat cleared up 3 days after I started taking penicillin. Why did I have to keep taking the antibiotic when I felt so much better?**

A Antibiotics, which are prescribed only for bacterial infections, can eliminate your symptoms within a few days. But some of the disease-causing bacteria survive in your body, ready to begin multiplying again if you stop taking the antibiotic too soon. For this reason, it is crucial that you take the full course that your doctor prescribes.

Q **My doctor would not prescribe an antibiotic for my cold. Why wouldn't she give me this relief?**

A Colds and most other respiratory infections are caused by viruses. Antibiotics are not effective against viral illnesses. In addition, you would be exposing yourself to the unnecessary risk of side effects such as an allergic reaction to the antibiotic and the destruction of helpful bacteria in your body, which could lead to other infections.

Q **I have been taking antibiotics for bronchitis for the past 10 days and now I have developed a vaginal yeast infection. Why?**

A Antibiotics sometimes destroy harmless bacteria that normally live in the body, primarily in the mouth, gastrointestinal tract, and vagina. When these friendly bacteria are destroyed, it opens the way for disease-causing organisms to take over and cause infections such as the yeast infection you have. This is why doctors are careful to prescribe antibiotics only when necessary.

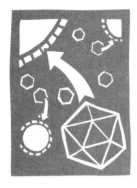

VIRUSES

VIRUSES CAUSE a wide range of illnesses, from the common cold to life-threatening diseases such as AIDS. Viruses are parasites – in order to survive and replicate, they must invade living cells and take over their internal processes. On their own, viruses are incapable of activities necessary for life, such as metabolism, growth, and reproduction.

Viruses live off all forms of life – animals, plants, and even bacteria. They are so small that most can only be seen with a powerful microscope. A single virus particle consists of genetic material (either DNA or RNA) encapsulated in a one- or two-layer protein shell. Some viruses are enclosed in another layer, called a viral envelope. Of all infectious agents, viruses have the fewest genes – the units of hereditary material. Some viruses have only three or four genes, compared with the tens of thousands that people have. This limited amount of genetic material and the inability to process nutrients make it necessary for viruses to hijack cells of other organisms (host cells) in order to survive.

HOW VIRUSES REPLICATE

Viruses use different strategies to make copies of themselves once they have invaded a cell, but the basic process of replication is shown below and at right. In order to multiply, viruses must use the reproductive and metabolic parts of living cells. This disrupts the normal functioning of cells and leads to the symptoms of disease. Some viruses, however, can be present in the body and not cause illness.

1 To reproduce, viruses first must gain entry to cells. Surface proteins on the shell of the virus or on its outer envelope attach to specific protein receptors on the surface of the host cell. Because different viruses bind to specific receptors on different types of cells, individual viruses may infect only certain organs in the body.

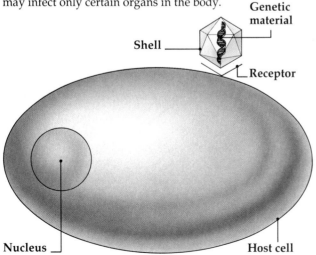

Genetic material

Shell

Receptor

Nucleus

Host cell

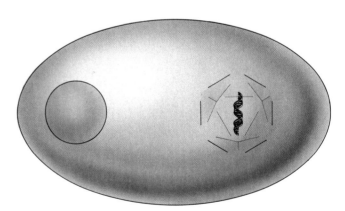

2 Once inside the cell, the viral shell falls apart or is broken down by enzymes (proteins that regulate the rate of chemical reactions in the body). The genetic material of the virus is released into the host cell.

3 The viral genetic material replicates, using enzymes inside the host cell. Larger viruses may contribute some of their own enzymes to boost the replication process.

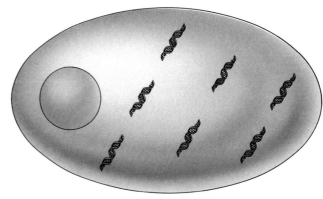

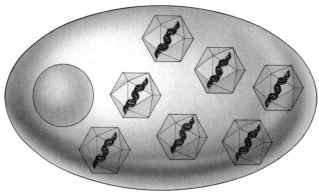

4 Each new copy of viral genetic material directs the formation of an outer protein shell. The genetic material and shell are assembled inside the host cell, forming complete virus particles.

5 The host cell becomes swollen with newly formed virus particles, which may eventually burst out of the cell, destroying it in the process.

6 Some viruses exit the host cell without destroying it. Instead, the virus forms a bud that breaks away from the cell, taking some of the cell membrane with it. An organism formed in this way is called an enveloped virus.

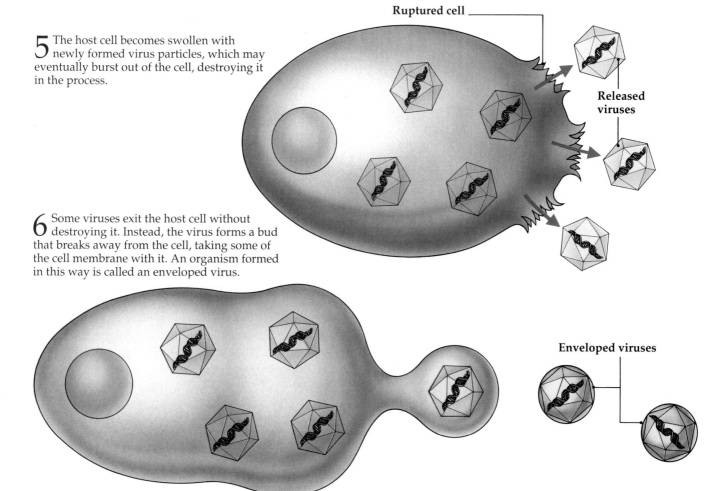

Ruptured cell

Released viruses

Enveloped viruses

STRUCTURES AND TYPES OF VIRUSES

All viruses are made of a symmetrical, outer protective layer of protein surrounding an inner core of genetic material. Viruses come in a variety of shapes and sizes, ranging from one millionth to one hundred thousandth of an inch in diameter. Viruses are assigned to groups based primarily on their structure. The most common virus families are listed below.

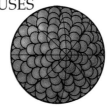 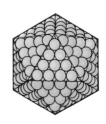 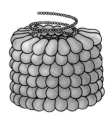

Shapes of viruses
The arrangement of the subunits of its outer shell determine a virus's shape. The three main structures are (from left to right) spherical, such as influenza viruses; 20-sided symmetrical solids, such as some viruses that cause respiratory and eye infections; and bullet-shaped, such as rabies viruses.

FAMILY	STRUCTURE	EXAMPLES OF CONDITIONS CAUSED
Adenoviruses	Medium-sized, 20-sided solids with spikes projecting from the corners	Respiratory and eye infections
Papovaviruses	Medium-sized, 20-sided solids	Warts on the hands, feet, genitals, anus, and occasionally inside the mouth and larynx
Herpesviruses	Large, enveloped, 20-sided solids	Cold sores, genital herpes, chickenpox, shingles, and infectious mononucleosis
Coronaviruses	Small spheres with projections	The common cold
Picornaviruses	Small, 20-sided solids	Polio, viral hepatitis, myocarditis, and aseptic meningitis; one group (rhinoviruses) causes colds
Rhabdoviruses	Bullet-shaped, enveloped particles with shells of subunits arranged in a spiral	Rabies
Reoviruses	Medium-sized, double-shelled, 20-sided solids	Mild respiratory infections; one group (rotaviruses) is a common cause of gastroenteritis
Orthomyxoviruses	Large, spherical, enveloped particles, covered with spikes	Influenza
Paramyxoviruses	Large, spherical, enveloped particles	Croup, measles, rubella (German measles), and mumps
Retroviruses	Spherical, enveloped particles covered with projections	AIDS and T cell leukemia

INSIDIOUS EFFECTS OF VIRUSES

Apart from the symptoms that viral infections produce, some viruses are thought to be factors in the development of other, noninfectious conditions. Research suggests that insulin-dependent diabetes may be caused by reactivation of a coxsackievirus later in life, after initial infection at a young age. This reactivation may provoke an immune response that destroys the insulin-producing cells of the pancreas. Another dangerous property of some viruses—called retroviruses—is the ability to integrate their own genetic material into the genetic material (DNA) of the host cell. This capability has the potential to deactivate a host-cell gene, alter its function, or even "switch on" a normally inactive gene. The effects of these mechanisms may contribute to the development of other diseases.

Viruses and oncogenes
When viral DNA incorporates itself into a cell and affects the genes that control cell growth or division, the result may be uncontrolled multiplication of the host cell, leading to the formation of a tumor.

HERPESVIRUS INFECTIONS

Herpesviruses are some of the most common and troublesome viruses. The group includes herpes simplex virus, varicella-zoster virus, Epstein-Barr virus, and cytomegalovirus. After the initial infection, herpesviruses are able to incorporate some of their genetic material into the nucleus of the host cell. Once inside the cell, the virus may lie dormant, avoiding detection by the immune system. Symptoms may recur if the virus is reactivated and multiplies inside cells. Doctors do not clearly understand what reactivates a virus.

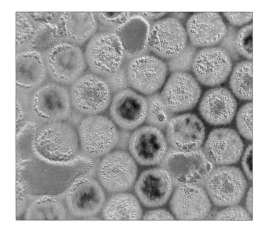

Shape of herpesviruses
All herpesviruses have the same basic shape. They are large, 20-sided, enveloped particles. The color-enhanced photograph at left (magnified 90,000 times) shows many herpes simplex virus particles. Herpesviruses contain DNA as their genetic material.

Herpes simplex virus
Herpes simplex virus causes infections usually characterized by blisterlike sores. Both the initial infection and reactivation of the virus cause sores to

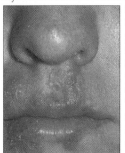

develop around the mouth (cold sores at left) or in the genital area. In more severe cases, the virus may cause herpetic whitlow (sores on the fingers) and keratoconjunctivitis, which affects the cornea and conjunctiva (the transparent membranes covering the white of the eye). Herpes simplex virus can also cause encephalitis (inflammation of the brain), which can be fatal if not treated.

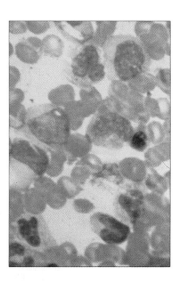

Epstein-Barr virus
Most infections with Epstein-Barr virus cause no symptoms, but in some cases the virus leads to infectious mononucleosis. This condition is characterized by fever, swollen glands, a sore throat, fatigue, and the presence of abnormal lymphocytes (purple-stained cells in the blood smear at left, magnified 1,000 times), which are a type of defensive white blood cell. The virus is a cause of Burkitt's lymphoma – a rare cancer of the lymph glands in the jaw.

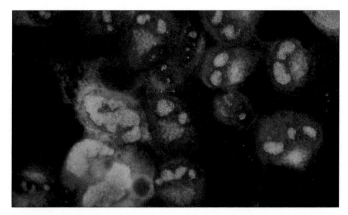

Cytomegalovirus
Cytomegalovirus, which means "big cell virus," makes infected cells grow larger. The infection is very common and occasionally causes symptoms similar to those of mononucleosis. The virus is a frequent cause of pneumonia in people undergoing bone marrow or organ transplantation. The photograph above (magnified 440 times) shows cells infected with cytomegalovirus (bright green ovals).

Varicella-zoster virus
Initial infection with the varicella-zoster virus causes chickenpox (varicella), a common childhood illness characterized by fever and a rash with blisters. The virus then remains dormant, seldom recurring. However, if the virus is reactivated, particularly in older people or in people whose immune systems are compromised, it causes a more severe illness called shingles (herpes zoster), which produces a rash such as that shown at right.

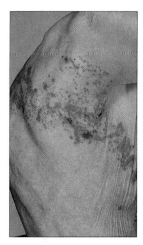

Genes that can be switched on in this way are called oncogenes. Some types of cancer may be caused by viruses. Studies show that women who have been exposed to strains of papillomavirus that cause genital warts have a greatly increased risk of cervical cancer. Other cancers associated with viruses include penile cancer, liver cancer, Burkitt's lymphoma, and T cell leukemia.

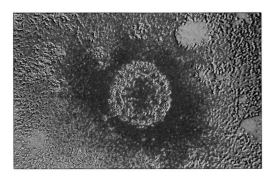

Hepatitis B virus
Hepatitis B virus (shown in the color-enhanced photograph above, magnified 500,000 times) is associated with hepatocellular carcinoma, a type of liver cancer. Viral DNA has been found integrated into the DNA of liver cells of people with the cancer.

SLOW VIRUS DISEASES

Slow virus diseases are a group of rare illnesses whose symptoms may not appear for months or even years after initial infection. Although they are called slow "virus" diseases, the causative agent has never been found. The disease-causing organism is thought to be a prion – a protein molecule that is smaller than even the smallest virus and is capable of replication. One slow virus disease, Creutzfeldt-Jakob syndrome, which affects the brain, has been transmitted during organ transplantation but doctors do not know how. Kuru, another rare slow virus disease, has been found only in a tribe of people living in New Guinea. Kuru is thought to be acquired from the cannibalistic ritual of eating the brains of dead relatives. Since this practice was stopped several years ago, the incidence of the disease has fallen sharply.

DISEASES ASSOCIATED WITH AIDS

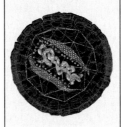

Infection with human immunodeficiency virus (HIV, above) eventually leads to the fatal disease AIDS. HIV infection weakens the immune system, paving the way for opportunistic infections, such as yeast infections, to get a foothold. The infection also increases a person's susceptibility to several types of cancer, such as Kaposi's sarcoma (a malignant tumor of the skin) and lymphoma of the brain, which causes dementia.

ASK YOUR DOCTOR
VIRAL ILLNESSES

Q Why must I be vaccinated only once or twice in my life against German measles but over and over against influenza?

A Most vaccines are made from modified live viruses that have been weakened so that they cannot cause disease. The modified viruses stimulate the immune system to become sensitized to the specific virus. This process enables the immune system to recognize the virus and be ready to destroy it should it enter the body a second time. However, some vaccines, such as the influenza vaccine, are made from killed viruses and provide immunity that lasts only a year.

Q Can I catch a viral infection from silverware or dishes used by infected people?

A Outside the body, most viruses can survive for only a very short time and are easily damaged by heat, dehydration, strong light, and disinfectants. Viruses and other disease organisms cannot be transmitted from one person to another on silverware or dishes as long as they have been washed after use. Sharing silverware at the same meal, however, may carry a slight risk of acquiring cold viruses.

Q I recently read in the newspaper that a person can die from measles? Is this true?

A Yes, but it is rare. In one in 1,000 cases, measles leads to encephalitis (inflammation of the brain), which can be fatal. Measles may also lead to bacterial lung or ear infections, which can be dangerous to children and to adults in poor health.

ANTIVIRAL DRUGS

To reproduce, most viruses must incorporate their own genetic material (DNA or RNA) into the genetic material in the nucleus of the host cell. As a result, a drug that injures a virus may also harm the host cell. The speed with which viruses are able to multiply is another problem. To be effective, antiviral drugs must be taken preventively or early in the course of an infection. Most antiviral drugs act by inhibiting viral replication. Zidovudine (AZT), which is taken by some people who are infected with HIV (the AIDS virus), and acyclovir (used for herpesvirus infections) work in this way (see below). Some antiviral drugs, such as amantadine, which is used to prevent influenza, actually keep viruses from penetrating host cells.

HOW SOME DRUGS SABOTAGE VIRAL REPLICATION

Both DNA and RNA consist of a chain of substances called nucleosides, of which there are five types – adenosine, guanosine, thymidine, cytidine, and uracil (which replaces thymidine in RNA). Antiviral drugs such as acyclovir and zidovudine are called nucleoside analogues because they have a structure very similar to a specific nucleoside. The virus mistakenly uses the drug instead of the real nucleoside, disrupting its replication process.

KEY	
Guanosine	Cytidine
Adenosine	Thymidine
Acyclovir	Uracil
	Zido-vudine

Acyclovir
The antiviral drug acyclovir, used to treat herpesvirus infections, has a structure very similar to the nucleoside guanosine.

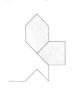

Guanosine   Acyclovir

Zidovudine
The antiviral drug zidovudine (AZT), used to treat HIV-infected people, has a structure similar to the nucleoside thymidine.

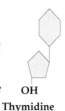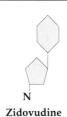

OH   N
Thymidine   Zidovudine

Herpesvirus replication without acyclovir
Because viral DNA contains the same four basic nucleosides as host cell DNA, a nucleoside of herpesvirus DNA can link onto any nucleoside of host cell DNA. The viral DNA is integrated into host cell DNA. The virus is then able to use host enzymes to replicate.

HIV replication without zidovudine
HIV contains RNA as its genetic material. Because host enzymes can act only on DNA, the virus first must convert its RNA into DNA using an enzyme called reverse transcriptase. The new viral DNA can then integrate into the host DNA and replicate.

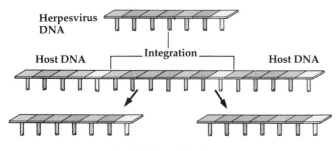

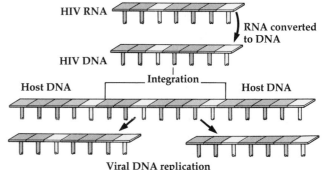

Herpesvirus replication with acyclovir
The herpesvirus is tricked into using acyclovir instead of guanosine. But acyclovir does not have the proper structure to link onto the next nucleoside of the host cell's DNA chain, preventing viral DNA integration and blocking the virus's ability to replicate.

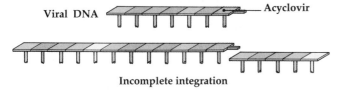

HIV replication with zidovudine
Zidovudine acts very early in the HIV replication cycle. As the virus converts viral RNA into DNA, reverse transcriptase is tricked into using zidovudine instead of thymidine. It is then unable to add the next nucleoside in the DNA sequence.

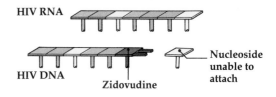

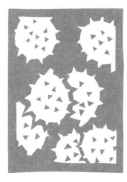

FUNGI

UNGI ARE SIMPLE parasitic life-forms. There are more than 100,000 different species, including molds, mildews, yeasts, and mushrooms. Many fungi are safe to ingest; yeasts are used in baking and brewing and we can eat some mushrooms. But some of these parasites are capable of causing disease.

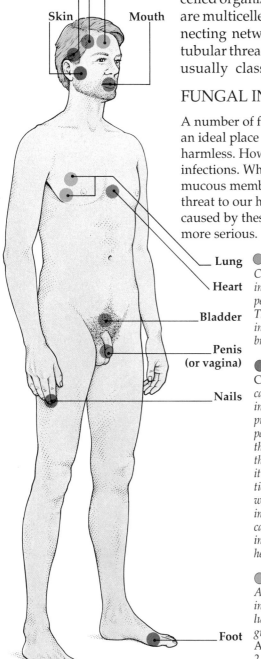

Scalp   Brain
Skin   Mouth

Lung
Heart

Bladder

Penis
(or vagina)

Nails

Foot

Some fungi, such as yeasts, are single-celled organisms. Others, such as molds, are multicelled and grow as an interconnecting network of branched chains of tubular threads called hyphae. Fungi are usually classified as a type of plant because, like plants, they have cell walls and they cannot move on their own. Unlike plants, however, they cannot manufacture their own food; they have to obtain their nutrients from other organisms, living or dead.

FUNGAL INFECTIONS

A number of fungi find the human body an ideal place to live and most of them are harmless. However, some can cause infections. When fungi attack the skin or mucous membranes, they are usually not a threat to our health. But internal infections caused by these organisms can often be more serious.

● Cryptococcosis
Cryptococcosis is an opportunistic infection – that is, it usually attacks people whose resistance is lowered. The fungus can initially cause lung infections, but may spread to the brain, causing meningitis.

● Candidiasis
Candida *organisms cause candidiasis, commonly called a yeast infection. Oral candidiasis (thrush) produces redness and whitish patches on the tongue and gums. In the vagina, candidiasis produces a thick, creamy discharge; on the penis, it causes itchy redness. Yeast infections often occur during treatment with antibiotics or in people whose immune systems are weakened. Occasionally, these infections can occur in the bloodstream, bladder, brain, or heart valves.*

● Aspergillosis
Aspergillosis is an opportunistic infection that usually occurs in the lungs. The color-enhanced photograph at right shows the fungus Aspergillus fumigatus *(magnified 2,400 times) forming spores.*

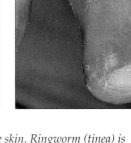

● Dermatophytosis
Dermatophytes infect the skin. Ringworm (tinea) is the most common of these infections and can affect the feet (athletes' foot, shown above right), nails, face, and scalp. An example of ringworm affecting the face is shown above left.

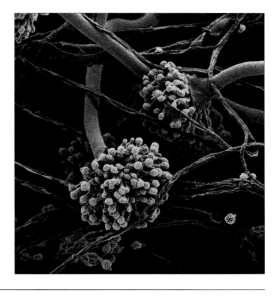

HOW FUNGI GROW

Fungi often have a two-stage life cycle. They may multiply sexually when two hyphae (tubular threads) of opposite sexes meet and pool their genetic material. Or they may grow asexually from a single spore to form a complex mass of hyphae, called a mycelium.

Sexual reproduction
Two hyphae of opposite sexes meet and form cells called gametes. The gametes fuse to form a zygote that contains their combined genetic material. The zygote germinates and produces spores that often spread to new sites.

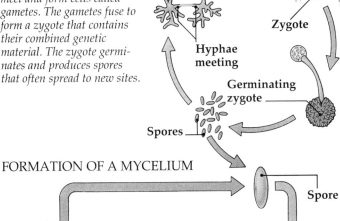

Gametes

Zygote

Hyphae meeting

Germinating zygote

Spores

FORMATION OF A MYCELIUM

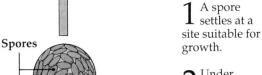

Spore

Spores

1 A spore settles at a site suitable for growth.

2 Under favorable conditions, such as having enough nutrients, the spore grows and divides.

4 Eventually, a complex network of hyphae – the mycelium – develops. The colony may start forming its own spores.

3 The fungi may continue to divide into branched chains of tubular threads called hyphae.

Hyphae

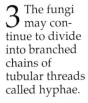

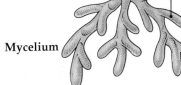

Mycelium

TREATING FUNGAL INFECTIONS

Fungal infections are more difficult to treat than bacterial infections. Fungal cells resemble human cells, so many substances that destroy the fungus can also damage body cells. Still, several safe antifungal drugs are available.

Nystatin is one of the oldest and most common treatments for mild candidiasis (a yeast infection). Amphotericin B may be used to treat more serious yeast infections and other internal fungal infections. Ketoconazole and miconazole are used to treat yeast infections. Ketoconazole is also used to treat ringworm. A new drug, fluconazole, is very effective in treating serious fungal infections such as cryptococcosis, which can affect the central nervous system. Antifungal drugs are taken as tablets, liquids, vaginal suppositories, ointments, or injections, depending on the type and site of infection. Antibiotics are effective in treating some fungal infections.

HEALTHY FUNGAL CELL

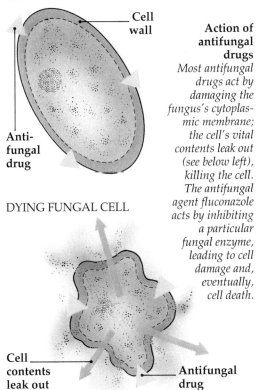

Cell wall

Antifungal drug

Action of antifungal drugs
Most antifungal drugs act by damaging the fungus's cytoplasmic membrane; the cell's vital contents leak out (see below left), killing the cell. The antifungal agent fluconazole acts by inhibiting a particular fungal enzyme, leading to cell damage and, eventually, cell death.

DYING FUNGAL CELL

Cell contents leak out

Antifungal drug

ANIMAL PARASITES

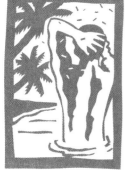

MANY DIFFERENT TYPES of animal parasites – ranging from tiny amebae to organisms such as worms that are visible to the naked eye – are capable of living in or on our bodies. In many cases, we hardly notice their presence, but some of these parasites can cause distressing symptoms and serious illnesses.

Plasmodium falciparum
(causes falciparum malaria)

Ingested red blood cells

Entamoeba histolytica
(causes amebiasis)

Giardia lamblia
(causes giardiasis)

Trichomonas vaginalis
(causes trichomoniasis)

Types of protozoa
Five different disease-causing protozoa are shown here. A protozoan differs from a bacterium in that it has a well-defined nucleus and no cell wall. Protozoa are much larger than bacteria and many are capable of movement. The organisms that cause giardiasis and trichomoniasis have long whiplike appendages (flagella) that they use to propel themselves. An Entamoeba histolytica *ameba moves by extending part of its body forward and then pulling the rest of itself in. Amebae are capable of ingesting food particles and red blood cells. They may also invade inflamed tissues.*

Trypanosoma cruzi
(causes Chagas' disease)

Protozoa, worms (helminths), and lice and mites (ectoparasites) make up the three main groups of animal parasites that can live on people.

PROTOZOA

Protozoa are microscopic, single-celled animals. They get their nourishment by scavenging for and ingesting small food particles and other microorganisms or by absorbing nutrients from their environment. Some protozoa invade human or animal cells as part of their life cycle.

Disease-causing protozoa

The few protozoa that cause disease in people fall into two main groups. Protozoa belonging to the first group spend part of their life cycle in people and another part in insects. When an insect bites a person, infectious protozoa can be passed either way between them. Diseases caused by these parasites are confined primarily to the tropics and subtropics. Worldwide, there are an estimated 110 million cases each year of malaria, the most prevalent of these diseases. Other such illnesses include sleeping sickness, which is transmitted by tsetse flies and occurs primarily in Africa; Chagas' disease, which occurs in South America; and leishmaniasis, a variety of diseases that affect the skin, mucous membranes, and internal organs. Leishmaniasis, which does not occur in the US, is transmitted by sandflies.

Protozoa belonging to the second group, which pass from person to person by means other than insect bites, are

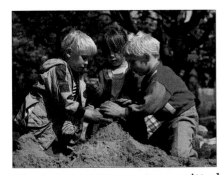

Giardiasis in children
This intestinal infection is common in pre-schoolers, particularly those who have close physical contact with many other children.

found throughout the world. Different protozoa in this group cause amebiasis and giardiasis, two intestinal infections that can cause severe diarrhea (see PROTOZOAL INFECTIONS on page 112), and trichomoniasis, a common sexually transmitted infection (see page 138). Other diseases in this group include toxoplasmosis (see page 56) and two so-called opportunistic infections (pneumocystis pneumonia and cryptosporidiosis) that primarily affect people with AIDS.

Malaria

Malaria is a protozoal disease that is transmitted by *Anopheles* mosquitoes. The disease occurs in parts of Mexico and the Caribbean, and much of South America, Africa, India, and Asia. Malaria produces a severe fever and chills and, in some cases, leads to potentially fatal complications. Approximately 1,000 cases of malaria are diagnosed in the US each year, mainly among immigrants or travelers who have returned from areas where the disease is present.

Travelers visiting those areas should take adequate precautions. Anyone who

LIFE CYCLE OF MALARIA PARASITE

Four different types of protozoa – called plasmodia – can cause malaria. The life cycle of one of the most common malaria-causing protozoa, *Plasmodium vivax*, is shown below. The others have similar life cycles, except for *Plasmodium falciparum*, which infects all red blood cells, not just imma-

ture cells. For this reason, the fever caused by *Plasmodium falciparum* is more irregular and prolonged. The illness, called falciparum malaria, is more severe and may affect the kidneys and brain. If not treated immediately, falciparum malaria can cause death within a few hours.

1 Infectious forms of the parasite, called sporozoites, enter the bloodstream from the saliva of a female *Anopheles* mosquito when it bites a person.

2 The parasites enter liver cells and multiply. Eventually, the liver cells release merozoites, another form of the parasite, into the bloodstream. A few parasites reenter or remain dormant in the liver.

3 The released merozoites invade immature red blood cells. Inside the cells, merozoites mature and multiply.

Sporozoites

Liver cell

Developing merozoites

Merozoites

Red blood cell

Male gametocyte

Female gametocyte

Merozoites

5 Some of the parasites develop into gametocytes, which can infect mosquitoes. Inside mosquitoes, gametocytes develop into forms that can infect people.

4 The parasites multiply rapidly in red blood cells, causing the cells to rupture and release large numbers of merozoites. The released parasites invade more red cells, which also rupture. This recurring cycle produces chills and a fever every other day.

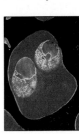

Two *Plasmodium falciparum* malaria parasites in a red blood cell (magnified 1,000 times).

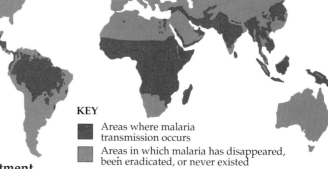

TRAVEL PRECAUTIONS AGAINST MALARIA

Malaria is the disease that poses the greatest threat to travelers to warm climates.

KEY

■ Areas where malaria transmission occurs

■ Areas in which malaria has disappeared, been eradicated, or never existed

Preventive drug treatment

Several weeks before traveling to any part of the world where malaria occurs, inform your doctor. The appropriate medication for you will depend on what area you intend to visit. Chloroquine is the best drug to use in some places, but malarial parasites in certain areas have become resistant to it, so other drugs are used instead. Your doctor will prescribe antimalarial medication for you to start taking a few days before arriving at your destination. In addition, you must continue taking the medication for 4 weeks after you return. Current information for travelers about malaria is available 24 hours a day from the Centers for Disease Control in Atlanta at (404) 639-1610.

Avoiding mosquito bites

Many factors determine the likelihood of being bitten by an infected mosquito in a part of the world where malaria exists. The risk is greatest in low-lying areas and less in areas at high altitudes. There is no malaria in places higher than 5,000 feet above sea level. Additionally, the risk is greater in rural areas than in cities. Mosquitoes are more likely to bite at dusk or at night than during the day. If you are staying in an area where the risk of infection exists, you should:

◆ Wear clothes that cover your feet, ankles, legs, and arms.

◆ Apply insect repellent to your face and hands.

◆ Sleep under a mosquito net or in an air-conditioned room with screens over the windows.

◆ Before going to sleep, use an insecticidal spray or burn a coil that releases insecticidal smoke into the room.

Remember that, in areas with malaria, most adults are immune to the disease and, therefore, they do not need to take precautions. Because you are not immune, the precautions are essential for you.

PROTOZOA-FIGHTING DRUGS

Several drugs are effective against the protozoal infections that commonly occur in the US. Metronidazole can be used to treat the intestinal infections amebiasis and giardiasis, and a sexually transmitted disease called trichomoniasis. A combination of pyrimethamine and sulfadiazine is used to treat toxoplasmosis. For malaria, chloroquine is the standard treatment, except in areas where the parasites are resistant to the drug. Other drugs, such as quinine, mefloquine, pyrimethamine, sulfadoxine, and tetracycline, are then used. The drugs work by killing the parasites directly. Side effects, particularly nausea, are common with all antiprotozoal drugs; treatment should be carefully monitored.

acquires an illness with a fever at any time up to 12 months after returning from such an area should notify his or her doctor. Malaria can be effectively treated once it is diagnosed.

Toxoplasmosis

Toxoplasmosis – caused by the protozoan *Toxoplasma gondii* – is a disease of ani-

mals that is frequently transmitted to people. People usually acquire toxoplasmosis by eating undercooked meat that has been infected by the protozoan. Infection can also occur by hand-to-mouth transmission if the hands become contaminated by infected cat feces. The infection usually produces no symptoms, but sometimes causes a fever and other symptoms resembling mononucleosis. In some cases, toxoplasmosis leads to serious complications, including damage to organs. Infection during pregnancy can cause a miscarriage or severe birth defects. Toxoplasmosis causes brain abscesses in people with AIDS.

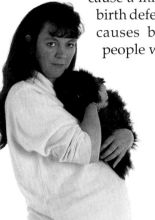

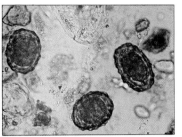

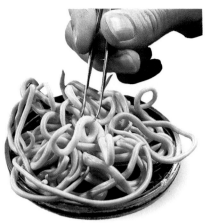

Cats and pregnancy
Because of the risk of toxoplasmosis, pregnant women should wash their hands after handling cats and should not change litter boxes, or should use gloves when doing so.

Common roundworm
The photograph at right shows several adult common roundworms, Ascaris lumbricoides. *A light infestation with these worms seldom provokes symptoms but sometimes causes mild abdominal pain. Occasionally, worms are eliminated in feces or vomit. Diagnosis is made when worm eggs (above, magnified 1,000 times) are found in the feces during microscopic examination. Infestations can be completely cleared up with a worm-fighting (anthelmintic) drug.*

LIFE CYCLE OF A ROUNDWORM

Toxocariasis is an infestation with the larvae of the roundworm *Toxocara canis,* which normally lives in dogs but can infest people, particularly children. Teach your children never to touch dog feces and make sure you have your dogs dewormed regularly.

1 A dog (often a puppy) harboring the worm in its digestive tract passes large numbers of worm eggs in its feces, which may contaminate the soil.

3 The eggs hatch in the intestines, freeing the larvae, which can then migrate through the tissues to organs such as the liver, lungs, and eyes. They can provoke allergic reactions such as asthma and may lead to serious complications, including loss of vision.

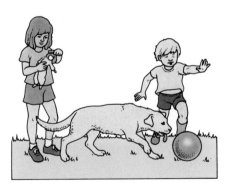

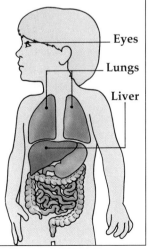

Eyes

Lungs

Liver

2 Children who play with an infested dog or with contaminated soil and who then put their fingers in their mouths may swallow some of the worm eggs.

WORMS

Several types of worms can live as parasites in people. They may infest the intestines, blood, lymphatic system, bile ducts, or organs such as the liver. Only a few kinds of worms are common in developed countries such as the US. In many cases, a worm infestation causes few, if any, symptoms; in fact, a person may have worms for years without realizing it. The discovery of an infestation can be alarming, but most worms can be easily eliminated with worm-fighting drugs called anthelmintics.

Parasitic worms fall into two main groups – cylindrically shaped worms called nematodes or roundworms, and flat-bodied worms called flatworms, which include tapeworms and flukes.

Roundworms

The common roundworm and the pinworm infest people in the US more frequently than any other type of worm. Both worms live in the intestines.

The adult common roundworm is nearly 10 inches long and about as thick as a pencil. Female worms produce eggs that are eliminated from the body in feces. If another person ingests these eggs – by eating contaminated food, for instance – the eggs will hatch into larvae that eventually settle and grow into adults in the person's intestines, setting up a new infestation.

Pinworms, which are less than a third of an inch long, primarily affect children. At night, the female adult worm crawls out of the intestines and lays eggs in the skin around the anus, causing severe itching. Pinworms can be eliminated easily with anthelmintic drugs. The whole family must be treated at the same time because the infestation can be passed among family members.

Toxocariasis and trichinosis are rare but potentially serious roundworm infections. The life cycle of the *Toxocara canis* roundworm is shown on page 57. Trichinosis is acquired by eating undercooked pork that contains larval cysts of the worm *Trichinella spiralis*. The infestation may cause symptoms such as fever and muscle aches as the larvae move through the body and settle in muscles. Occasionally, people become seriously ill with trichinosis.

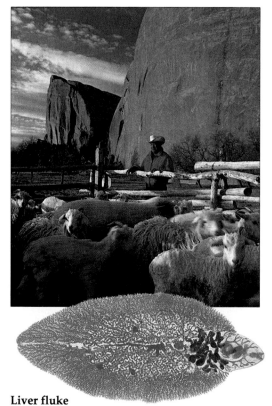

Liver fluke
This parasitic flatworm (above, magnified two times) normally infests sheep but can be transmitted to humans who eat plants that have been contaminated by larval forms of the fluke.

ANTHELMINTIC DRUGS

Several drugs – such as mebendazole, thiabendazole, ivermectin, pyrantel, and niclosamide – may be used to treat worm infestations. The drugs either kill or paralyze the worms. In the intestines, the drugs loosen the worms' grip on the intestinal wall so they can be eliminated from the body in feces. In other tissues, the drugs make the worms vulnerable to attack by the immune system. Anthelmintic drugs sometimes produce side effects, including nausea, vomiting, and abdominal pain.

Hookworms are a common cause of anemia in people who live in the tropics. They are acquired by walking barefoot on soil contaminated with hookworm eggs and larvae.

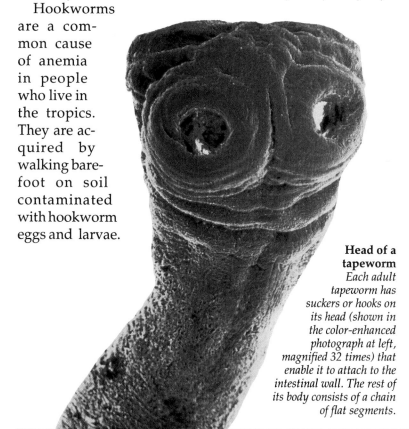

Head of a tapeworm
Each adult tapeworm has suckers or hooks on its head (shown in the color-enhanced photograph at left, magnified 32 times) that enable it to attach to the intestinal wall. The rest of its body consists of a chain of flat segments.

Tapeworms and flukes

Tapeworms and flukes, which are rare in the US, spend part of their lives in humans and part in animals.

Three different types of large tapeworms – acquired by eating undercooked beef, pork, or fish – can infest people. These infestations usually produce only mild symptoms, but segments of a tapeworm may detach and appear in the feces. In rare cases, fish tapeworms cause anemia. Anthelmintic drugs are effective in eradicating tapeworms.

The liver fluke, found mainly in China, causes symptoms such as jaundice (yellowing of the skin and whites of the eyes) when it settles inside the bile ducts of the liver. In many tropical countries, a fluke infestation called schistosomiasis is a major health problem. Schistosomiasis, which spreads through contact with contaminated water, afflicts more than 200 million people worldwide.

LIFE CYCLE OF TAPEWORMS

Humans can be primary hosts for three types of worms for which cattle, pigs, and fish are intermediate hosts – that is, the animals carry an immature form of the worm (see below). Interruptions in the tapeworm's life cycle – such as sanitary sewage disposal – can prevent these infestations.

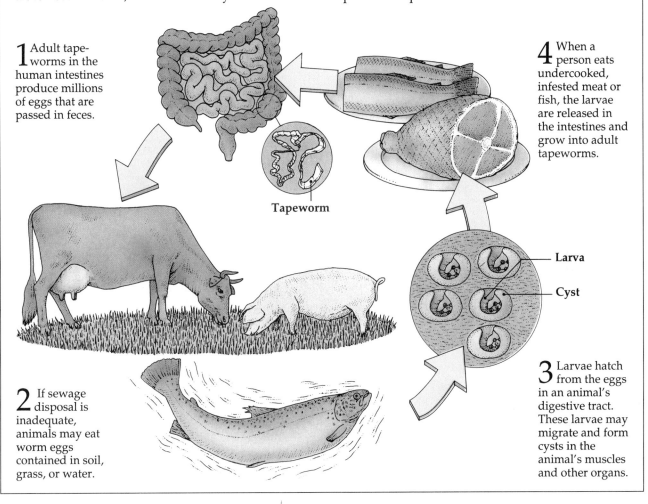

1 Adult tapeworms in the human intestines produce millions of eggs that are passed in feces.

Tapeworm

4 When a person eats undercooked, infested meat or fish, the larvae are released in the intestines and grow into adult tapeworms.

Larva

Cyst

2 If sewage disposal is inadequate, animals may eat worm eggs contained in soil, grass, or water.

3 Larvae hatch from the eggs in an animal's digestive tract. These larvae may migrate and form cysts in the animal's muscles and other organs.

Scabies mite
This tiny animal (right, magnified 60 times) has a round body and eight legs. It is about 1/50 of an inch long.

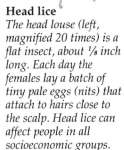

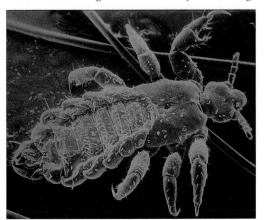

Head lice
The head louse (left, magnified 20 times) is a flat insect, about 1/8 inch long. Each day the females lay a batch of tiny pale eggs (nits) that attach to hairs close to the scalp. Head lice can affect people in all socioeconomic groups.

LICE AND MITES

Head lice, body lice, and crab (or pubic) lice are small, wingless insects that feed on human blood (see SKIN INFESTATIONS on page 124 and CRAB LICE on page 134).

The scabies mite, which resembles a tiny spider, burrows into the skin and lays its eggs, causing itching and inflammation. The mite is usually found on the wrists, genitals, or areas between the fingers or on the trunk. Scabies seems to occur in epidemic cycles. Both lice and mite infestations are easily treated with insecticidal shampoos or lotions.

CHAPTER THREE

FIGHTING INFECTION

YOUNG PEOPLE in the US today are virtually free from the danger of life-threatening infectious diseases, with the notable exception of AIDS. Until well into this century, infectious diseases were the most common cause of death. But, in developed countries like the US, this devastating pattern has been broken by improved public health measures and advances in medicine and technology. Still, infectious diseases remain a major killer in many parts of the world. This chapter describes the many ways we can prevent and protect ourselves against infections on both the individual and community levels. The first section highlights our most powerful resource – the body's own defenses – provided by an intricate and highly efficient immune system. As long as we stay well nourished and healthy, our immune system can cope with all but the most harmful invading organisms. In fact, it is the immune system that makes it actually beneficial for us to acquire and overcome certain infections, such as chickenpox, early in life rather than later, when they tend to be more serious. But even a healthy immune system provides only partial protection against certain dangerous organisms. To overcome these limitations, scientists have devised ways of har-

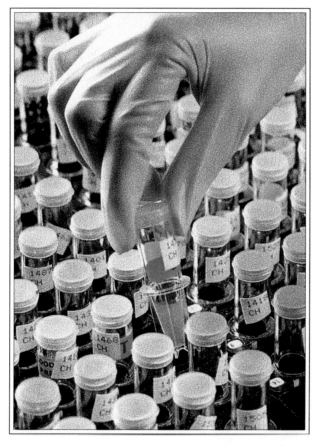

nessing the power of the immune system to fight off infections it otherwise could not cope with. Through widespread immunization, the incidence of life-threatening infections such as polio and diphtheria, as well as measles and mumps, has been dramatically reduced. The objective of immunization is to protect the individual, but immunization of large numbers of people protects the community as well. If a large proportion of a population is immune to a particular disease, it is unlikely that an epidemic will occur. In the US, we take it for granted that the food we eat, the water we drink, and the air we breathe is free from dangerous microbes. Before the emergence of AIDS, we had come to expect that public health measures would limit the extent of a serious epidemic. For the most part, our sophisticated monitoring and intervention system does provide successful disease control. The section on public health in this chapter explains some of the fundamental forces at work in this system. The development of antibiotics and other disease-fighting drugs has also played a significant role in the fight against infections. But before an infection can be treated, it must first be identified. How infectious diseases are diagnosed is explained in the final section of the chapter.

YOUR BODY'S DEFENSES

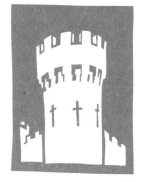

YOUR BODY IS CONSTANTLY threatened by millions of microorganisms and must therefore have effective defenses to protect itself. The body's ability to resist harm from microorganisms and damaging toxins is called immunity. It is the immune system that provides your body with a wide variety of mechanisms – both internal and external – to fight off disease-causing organisms.

Your immune system is divided into two main parts. One part is the nonspecific immune system you were born with. It is referred to as nonspecific because it responds in the same way to all invading organisms. This part of the immune system provides a variety of physical and chemical barriers against infection (see below) and is made up of many white blood cells that fight attacking organisms. The inflammatory response (see page 21) is a function of this system.

PHYSICAL AND CHEMICAL BARRIERS TO INFECTION

Physical barriers such as the skin, and chemical barriers such as tears, destroy most disease organisms before they can enter the body and cause harm.

Respiratory tract
Cells that line your respiratory tract secrete mucus that traps microbes. Mucus and microbes are swept out by cilia – hairlike extensions of the cells. Below is a color-enhanced photograph (magnified 500 times) showing mucus cells (purple) and cilia (orange).

Tears
Tears wash away disease organisms and, like sweat and saliva, they contain enzymes that destroy the germs.

Nose
Hairs in the nose trap microorganisms. The sneeze reflex helps to expel them. Nasal secretions contain enzymes that destroy germs.

Saliva
Saliva, like sweat and tears, contains enzymes that destroy disease organisms.

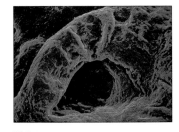

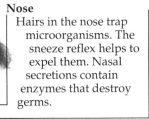

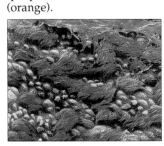

Skin
The skin is a highly effective barrier against germs. Oil glands in the skin secrete sebum, an acidic lubricating substance that is toxic to many bacteria. Sweat glands (such as the one shown in the color-enhanced photograph above, magnified 900 times) secrete microbe-destroying enzymes.

Stomach acid
In the stomach, hydrochloric acid occurs naturally and is toxic to many organisms.

Protective bacteria
Harmless bacteria in the vagina and the urethra compete with invading organisms and help protect us from disease.

The second part of your immune system, the adaptive immune system, identifies specific disease organisms and produces antibodies to attack them. Some cells can "remember" proteins (antigens) on the surface of organisms they have met, enabling them to respond rapidly and effectively to a repeat encounter.

ORGANS OF THE IMMUNE SYSTEM

A number of organs – including the bone marrow, tonsils, adenoids, spleen, lymph nodes and lymphatic vessels, and blood vessels – are involved in the functioning of the immune system.

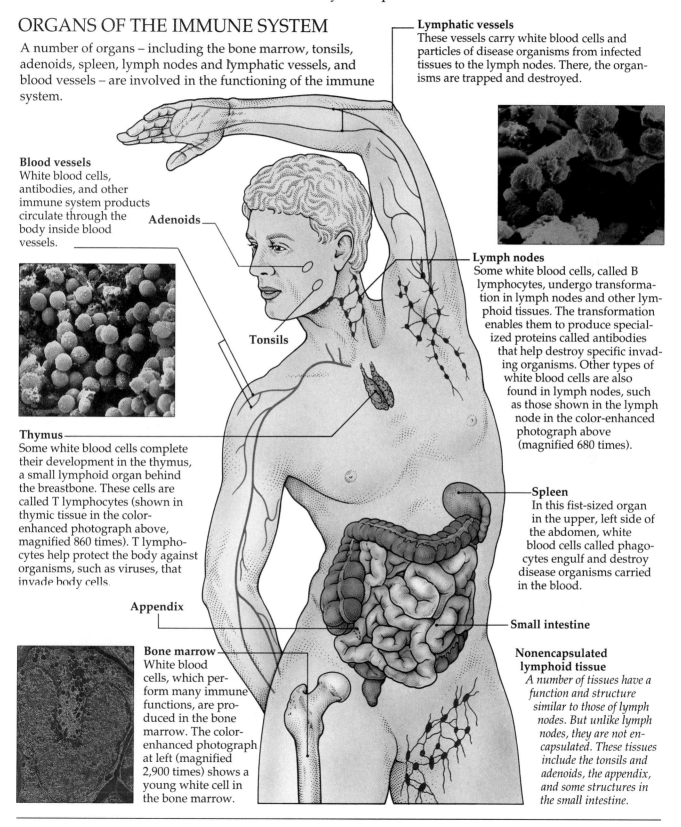

Lymphatic vessels
These vessels carry white blood cells and particles of disease organisms from infected tissues to the lymph nodes. There, the organisms are trapped and destroyed.

Blood vessels
White blood cells, antibodies, and other immune system products circulate through the body inside blood vessels.

Adenoids

Tonsils

Lymph nodes
Some white blood cells, called B lymphocytes, undergo transformation in lymph nodes and other lymphoid tissues. The transformation enables them to produce specialized proteins called antibodies that help destroy specific invading organisms. Other types of white blood cells are also found in lymph nodes, such as those shown in the lymph node in the color-enhanced photograph above (magnified 680 times).

Thymus
Some white blood cells complete their development in the thymus, a small lymphoid organ behind the breastbone. These cells are called T lymphocytes (shown in thymic tissue in the color-enhanced photograph above, magnified 860 times). T lymphocytes help protect the body against organisms, such as viruses, that invade body cells.

Spleen
In this fist-sized organ in the upper, left side of the abdomen, white blood cells called phagocytes engulf and destroy disease organisms carried in the blood.

Appendix

Small intestine

Bone marrow
White blood cells, which perform many immune functions, are produced in the bone marrow. The color-enhanced photograph at left (magnified 2,900 times) shows a young white cell in the bone marrow.

Nonencapsulated lymphoid tissue
A number of tissues have a function and structure similar to those of lymph nodes. But unlike lymph nodes, they are not encapsulated. These tissues include the tonsils and adenoids, the appendix, and some structures in the small intestine.

YOUR BODY'S RESPONSES TO INFECTION

Once disease-causing organisms enter the body, numerous defenses involving various types of white blood cells take action. These defensive responses are illustrated below.

FIRST LINE OF DEFENSE

Several types of white blood cells travel to the site of infection to prevent the invaders from advancing further. These white blood cells are cells of the nonspecific immune system. They respond to all invading organisms in the same way.

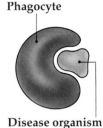
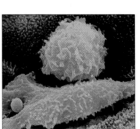

Phagocyte

Disease organism

Cells that "eat" bacteria
White blood cells called phagocytes – part of the first line of defense – travel to the site of infection, where they engulf and destroy invading disease organisms and then die. Large numbers of dead neutrophils (one type of phagocyte) form part of the substance known as pus. Another, larger type of phagocyte (shown in the color-enhanced photograph above, magnified 1,300 times), moves in to clean up the debris left by the neutrophils.

Natural killer cells
Natural killer cells are white blood cells that target and destroy invading organisms as well as cancer cells. They accomplish this destruction by releasing poisonous chemicals.

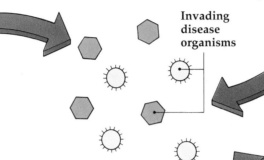

Invading disease organisms

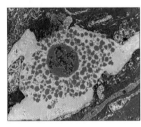

Cells that cause inflammation
Some white blood cells release chemicals at the site where the disease organism has entered the body, triggering the inflammatory response (see page 21). Chemical-releasing cells include mast cells (such as the one shown in the color-enhanced photograph above, magnified 1,300 times) and eosinophils (such as the one shown in the color-enhanced photograph at right, magnified 2,600 times).

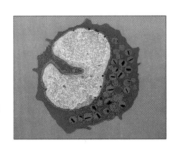

Interferons
Proteins called interferons are produced when cells are invaded by viruses. Interferons stimulate other cells to produce proteins that prevent the viruses from reproducing in the body.

THE COMPLEMENT SYSTEM

The complement system consists of about 25 inactive proteins that circulate in the blood. They are activated when the immune system makes antibodies to attack specific disease organisms. The proteins attach to the organism's surface and penetrate its membrane. Fluid rushes in and the organism bursts. The presence of disease organisms can also directly activate the complement system, which then triggers the inflammatory response and calls in the phagocytes, the engulfing destroyers.

1
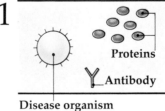
Proteins
Antibody
Disease organism

2
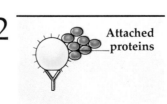
Attached proteins

3 **Dying organism**
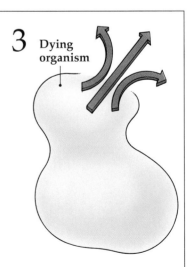

SECOND LINE OF DEFENSE

If disease organisms get past the first line of defense, more sophisticated cells move into action. They can identify specific invaders and tailor their attack accord-ingly. These "smart" cells make up the adaptive immune system, which has two divisions – one driven by antibodies and one driven by specialized blood cells.

ANTIBODY DEFENSES

B lymphocytes
Each B lymphocyte recognizes a particular disease organism. When B cells identify specific organisms, they multiply rapidly, turning themselves into plasma cells in the process. Plasma cells mass-produce unique proteins called antibodies, which seek out specific organisms and destroy them.

Memory B cells
After an infection, some B lymphocytes become memory cells. If the same disease organisms invade again, the memory B cells quickly manufacture antibodies to stop them.

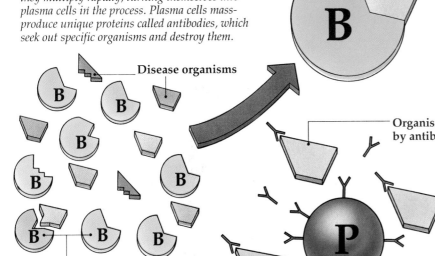

Recognition
Memory cells
Plasma cells
Disease organisms
Organism attacked by antibody
Antibodies
B lymphocytes

CELLULAR DEFENSES

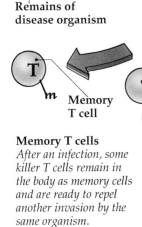

Killer T cell
Remains of disease organism
Memory T cell

Memory T cells
After an infection, some killer T cells remain in the body as memory cells and are ready to repel another invasion by the same organism.

Lymphokine

T lymphocytes
T lymphocytes (such as the one shown in the color-enhanced photograph below, magnified 2,300 times) protect us from disease organisms that invade body cells. They also fight cancer cells.

Killer T cells
When a killer T cell recognizes the remains of a disease organism that has been destroyed by a phagocyte, it immediately starts to multiply. Newly formed T cells seek out infected body cells, and, using potent proteins called lymphokines, destroy the invaders. But in the process, the infected cells themselves are also destroyed. Killer T cells destroy cancer cells too.

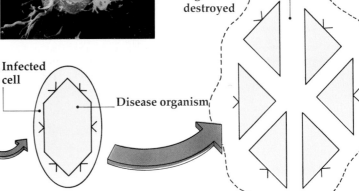

Cell and organism destroyed
Infected cell
Disease organism

MONITOR YOUR SYMPTOMS

FEVER

A fever – an abnormally high body temperature – is one of the signs that your body is fighting infection. You may feel just hot or you may feel shivery, hot, and sweaty – and you feel sick. Consult this chart if you have a temperature of 100°F (38°C) or above. Call your doctor at once if your temperature rises above 104°F (40°C) or remains at 100°F or higher for longer than 48 hours.

CONSULT YOUR DOCTOR WITHOUT DELAY!

Pneumonia or bronchitis may be the cause of your cough and other symptoms.

Action Your doctor will probably prescribe antibiotics and tell you to drink fluids and take a nonsteroidal anti-inflammatory drug, such as aspirin. Children should be given an aspirin substitute, not aspirin.

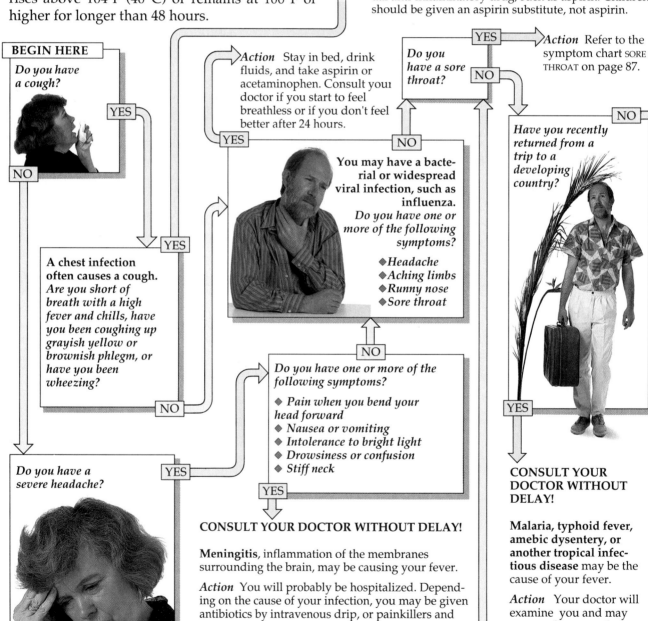

BEGIN HERE

Do you have a cough? YES / NO

Action Stay in bed, drink fluids, and take aspirin or acetaminophen. Consult your doctor if you start to feel breathless or if you don't feel better after 24 hours.

Do you have a sore throat? YES / NO

Action Refer to the symptom chart SORE THROAT on page 87.

You may have a bacterial or widespread viral infection, such as influenza.
Do you have one or more of the following symptoms?

◆ *Headache*
◆ *Aching limbs*
◆ *Runny nose*
◆ *Sore throat*

A chest infection often causes a cough. *Are you short of breath with a high fever and chills, have you been coughing up grayish yellow or brownish phlegm, or have you been wheezing?* YES / NO

Have you recently returned from a trip to a developing country? NO / YES

Do you have one or more of the following symptoms?

◆ *Pain when you bend your head forward*
◆ *Nausea or vomiting*
◆ *Intolerance to bright light*
◆ *Drowsiness or confusion*
◆ *Stiff neck*

Do you have a severe headache? YES / NO

CONSULT YOUR DOCTOR WITHOUT DELAY!

Meningitis, inflammation of the membranes surrounding the brain, may be causing your fever.

Action You will probably be hospitalized. Depending on the cause of your infection, you may be given antibiotics by intravenous drip, or painkillers and intravenous fluids. Bacterial meningitis is a life-threatening infection that requires immediate treatment with antibiotics.

CONSULT YOUR DOCTOR WITHOUT DELAY!

Malaria, typhoid fever, amebic dysentery, or another tropical infectious disease may be the cause of your fever.

Action Your doctor will examine you and may arrange for you to have blood and stool tests. Treatment will depend on the diagnosis.

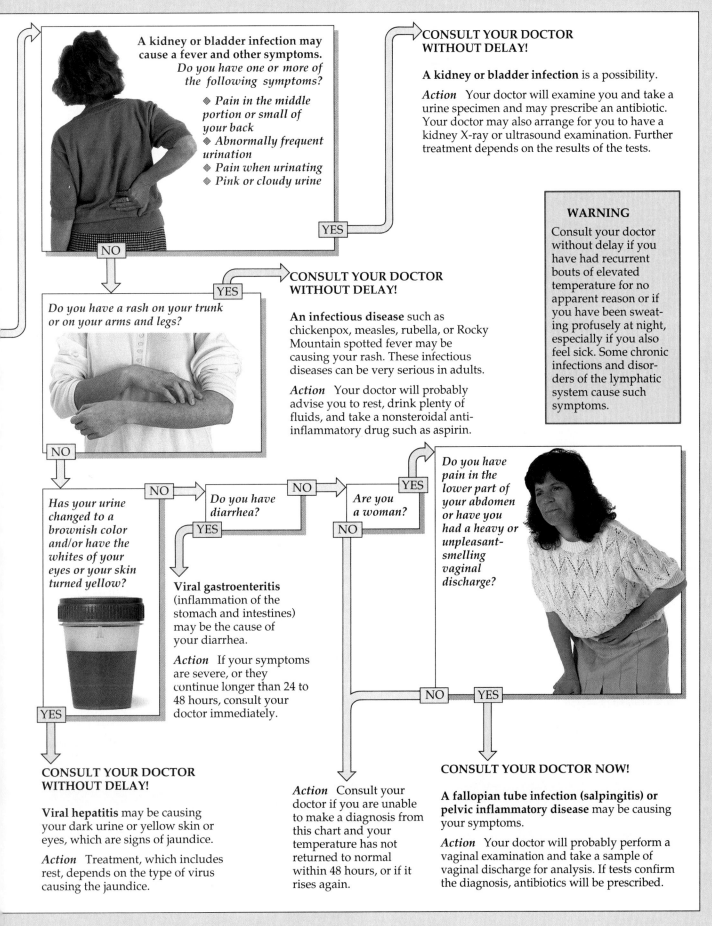

A kidney or bladder infection may cause a fever and other symptoms. *Do you have one or more of the following symptoms?*

◆ *Pain in the middle portion or small of your back*
◆ *Abnormally frequent urination*
◆ *Pain when urinating*
◆ *Pink or cloudy urine*

NO

YES

CONSULT YOUR DOCTOR WITHOUT DELAY!

A kidney or bladder infection is a possibility.

Action Your doctor will examine you and take a urine specimen and may prescribe an antibiotic. Your doctor may also arrange for you to have a kidney X-ray or ultrasound examination. Further treatment depends on the results of the tests.

WARNING

Consult your doctor without delay if you have had recurrent bouts of elevated temperature for no apparent reason or if you have been sweating profusely at night, especially if you also feel sick. Some chronic infections and disorders of the lymphatic system cause such symptoms.

YES

Do you have a rash on your trunk or on your arms and legs?

NO

CONSULT YOUR DOCTOR WITHOUT DELAY!

An infectious disease such as chickenpox, measles, rubella, or Rocky Mountain spotted fever may be causing your rash. These infectious diseases can be very serious in adults.

Action Your doctor will probably advise you to rest, drink plenty of fluids, and take a nonsteroidal anti-inflammatory drug such as aspirin.

Has your urine changed to a brownish color and/or have the whites of your eyes or your skin turned yellow?

NO

Do you have diarrhea?

NO

Are you a woman?

YES

Do you have pain in the lower part of your abdomen or have you had a heavy or unpleasant-smelling vaginal discharge?

YES

NO

YES

Viral gastroenteritis (inflammation of the stomach and intestines) may be the cause of your diarrhea.

Action If your symptoms are severe, or they continue longer than 24 to 48 hours, consult your doctor immediately.

NO   **YES**

YES

CONSULT YOUR DOCTOR WITHOUT DELAY!

Viral hepatitis may be causing your dark urine or yellow skin or eyes, which are signs of jaundice.

Action Treatment, which includes rest, depends on the type of virus causing the jaundice.

Action Consult your doctor if you are unable to make a diagnosis from this chart and your temperature has not returned to normal within 48 hours, or if it rises again.

CONSULT YOUR DOCTOR NOW!

A fallopian tube infection (salpingitis) or pelvic inflammatory disease may be causing your symptoms.

Action Your doctor will probably perform a vaginal examination and take a sample of vaginal discharge for analysis. If tests confirm the diagnosis, antibiotics will be prescribed.

PUBLIC HEALTH

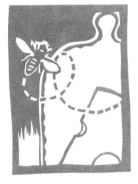

T HE DECLINE in the incidence of life-threatening infections is more the result of improved public health and sanitation than of antibiotics. Clean water supplies, adequate sewage treatment, sanitary handling of food and milk, and widespread immunization have eliminated many infectious diseases in the US, including typhoid fever, cholera, polio, and diphtheria.

Because of public health measures in the 20th century, infectious diseases are no longer the number one killer in the US.

SAFEGUARDING PUBLIC HEALTH

The US Department of Health and Human Services oversees research to detect the causes of disease and implements health education and disease prevention programs. The Public Health Service, a division of the department, carries out health policies set by the government. Two branches of the Public Health Service – the Centers for Disease Control and the Food and Drug Administration – play critical roles in controlling the spread of infectious diseases.

Food and Drug Administration

The Food and Drug Administration (FDA) administers federal laws designed to ensure the purity of food, the safety and effectiveness of drugs and medical devices, and the safety of cosmetics. The FDA is also concerned with the accuracy of labels and safety and honesty in product packaging. The FDA routinely monitors the nation's blood banks to ensure that blood is being properly screened for disease organisms. The agency also promotes sanitary conditions in public eating places and inspects food processing and drug manufacturing plants. Companies may be ordered to recall or stop producing products found to be harmful.

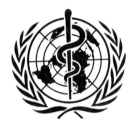

World Health Organization
The World Health Organization (WHO) was established in 1948 as an agency of the United Nations. It has instituted effective programs on a global scale to control or eradicate many infectious diseases, notably smallpox, tuberculosis, and malaria. WHO gathers information worldwide on communicable diseases, compiles health statistics, and provides international health standards and guidelines. WHO's current global health campaign is called "Health for All by the Year 2000."

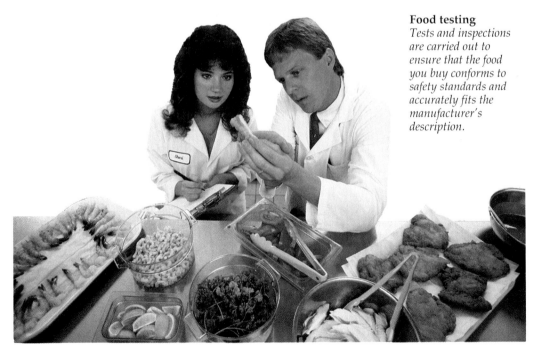

Food testing
Tests and inspections are carried out to ensure that the food you buy conforms to safety standards and accurately fits the manufacturer's description.

FOOD REGULATIONS

Public health regulations issued by the FDA, the US Department of Agriculture, and state and local health departments safeguard the food we buy. These measures ensure healthful practices at all stages of the preparation, manufacture, packaging, storage, and distribution of food. Food retailers are subject to regular state and local health authority inspections. A retailer who is found to be violating any of the regulations can be prosecuted. Restaurants are licensed and inspected by local health authorities.

Meat inspection

Meat is inspected at every stage of its production, from farm to store, to make sure that it is safe to eat. At the slaughterhouse, inspectors check carcasses thoroughly for signs of infection or parasites, such as larvae of beef tapeworms and pork roundworms.

Meat must be refrigerated at a specific temperature until it is processed or sold. Inspectors regularly check thermometers in refrigerators and freezers to make sure they are accurate to within 3°F. Bacteria can multiply when the temperature rises even a few degrees.

Processed and cooked meat
Processed and cooked meat or meat products must be cooked so that all parts of the food are heated to a temperature that destroys disease-causing organisms.

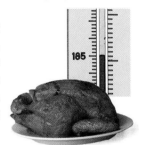

HYGIENE FOR FOOD HANDLERS

To prevent the spread of infectious diseases, strict regulations govern the preparation and sale of food. No one who is infected with a disease, or who has boils, sores, or an infected wound, is allowed to work in a food processing plant or retail outlet. If you are involved in any stage of food preparation, you must follow these rules:

◆ Wear clean outer garments.

◆ Wash your hands thoroughly with soap and water before starting work, each time your hands get dirty, and when you leave the work area.

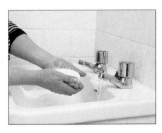

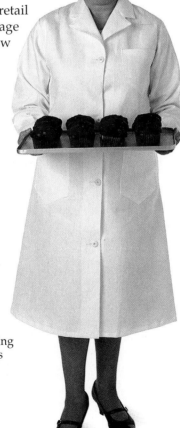

◆ Never eat, drink, smoke, or store clothing in areas where food is exposed or where utensils are washed.

◆ Wear a hair net, headband, cap, or other hair restraint.

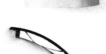

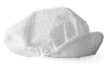

◆ Remove all jewelry that cannot be cleaned adequately.

◆ Make sure that any gloves used for handling food are kept clean and sanitary and are impermeable to water.

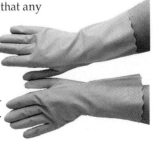

◆ Take any other necessary precautions to avoid contaminating food with germs or foreign substances, including perspiration, cosmetics, or chemicals.

SANITATION

Untreated sewage and impure water provide ideal environments for bacteria to live and multiply in. They also provide a route of transmission for infectious diseases such as typhoid fever, cholera, hepatitis, and dysentery. Pure water and safe sewage treatment play major roles in controlling the spread of disease. Human feces contain harmful microorganisms – including bacteria, viruses, and protozoa – that cause a wide range of diseases. Infections can spread when wastes contaminate our food or water supply. Boiling is recommended whenever the purity of drinking water is in question. Safe sewage treatment requires:

◆ No direct human contact with feces
◆ No contamination of water used for drinking or washing
◆ No access by animals or insects to fecal material
◆ No contact between feces and food

AIR CONDITIONING

Legionella pneumophila is the bacterium responsible for legionnaires' disease – a type of pneumonia that first came to public attention during an outbreak in Philadelphia in August 1976. Almost all of the people afflicted had attended an American Legion convention at a Philadelphia hotel. Since then, there have been many other reported cases of legionnaires' disease that have been linked to particular buildings. Evidence indicates that the disease is spread by inhaling airborne, infected particles rather than by person-to-person contact. Air-conditioning cooling towers and condensers that work by evaporation have now been identified as breeding places of the bacteria.

HOW IS SEWAGE PROCESSED?

Today's drainage systems and sewage plants provide safe processing of feces and other waste materials, as described below.

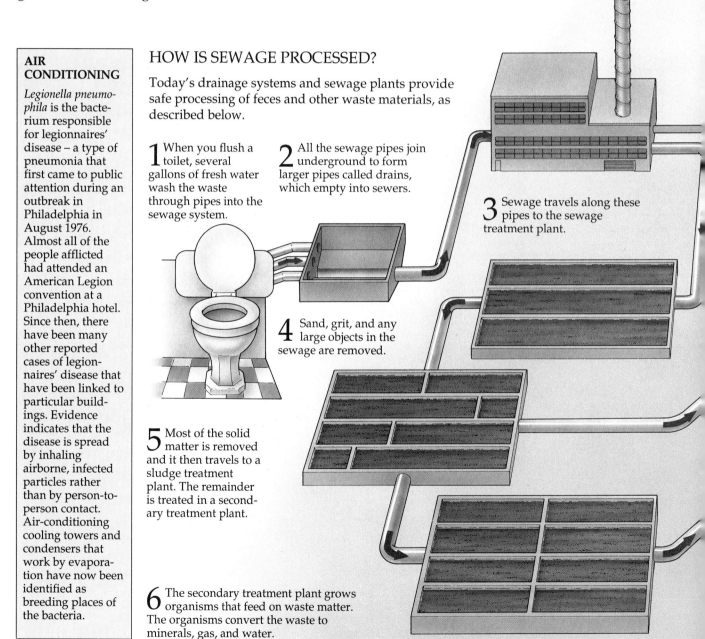

1 When you flush a toilet, several gallons of fresh water wash the waste through pipes into the sewage system.

2 All the sewage pipes join underground to form larger pipes called drains, which empty into sewers.

3 Sewage travels along these pipes to the sewage treatment plant.

4 Sand, grit, and any large objects in the sewage are removed.

5 Most of the solid matter is removed and it then travels to a sludge treatment plant. The remainder is treated in a secondary treatment plant.

6 The secondary treatment plant grows organisms that feed on waste matter. The organisms convert the waste to minerals, gas, and water.

CLEAN WATER SUPPLIES

We get our water from rain, from natural bodies of water such as lakes, rivers, and oceans, and from wells. Water should be tasteless, colorless, free of harmful organisms and chemicals, and clear. To meet these requirements, particles are removed through filtration and sedimentation, and the water is purified with chlorine or other disinfectants. Despite concern about the health effects of chlorine, it remains the most effective germ-killing agent. Irradiation and heat treatment are used to inactivate viruses that may be present in water. These measures provide us with a safe water supply.

Many disease organisms can live in water
Water is easily contaminated by human and animal feces and can carry harmful organisms such as bacteria, viruses, and parasites. Boiling is a simple way to purify water but is unnecessary in the US unless the water supply has been disrupted.

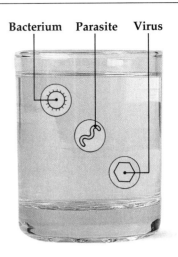

Bacterium   Parasite   Virus

7 The sludge is transferred to digestion tanks (below) where other microorganisms destroy the sewage materials and convert them to methane and other gases. The gas is used to fuel the electricity generator (left) that runs the sewage plant.

8 The remaining sludge is passed into open tanks. More gas is given off and the sludge settles, providing water and a thicker sludge.

9 The thick sludge is then used as landfill in strip-mining areas (below) or disposed of in other ways.

10 The waste water is filtered and treated with chemicals before it is released into a river, lake, or ocean.

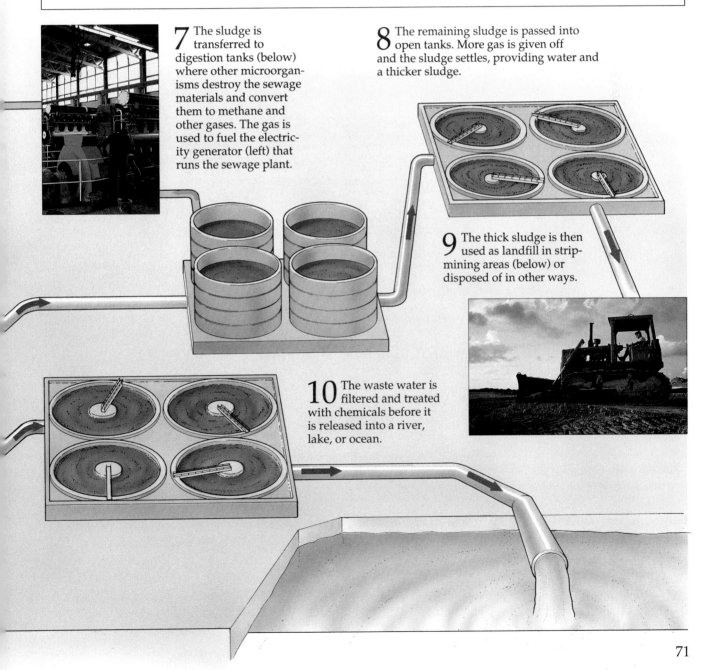

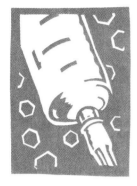

IMMUNIZATION

SOME INFECTIOUS DISEASES occur only once in a person's life because the body's immune system retains a memory of the disease and is ready to fight any subsequent infection by the same organism. The duration of this disease-induced immunity varies, but it can last a lifetime. Immunization is the process by which immunity to diseases that are potentially life-threatening is induced artificially.

TYPES OF IMMUNIZATION

Active immunization involves administering altered or killed forms of a disease organism, which stimulates the immune system the same way a true infection would. Passive immunization relies on the introduction of antibodies produced by people who have recovered from disease.

ACTIVE IMMUNIZATION

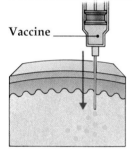

Vaccine

1 A person is injected with a vaccine containing killed or modified noninfectious forms of an organism.

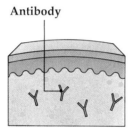

Antibody

2 The vaccine stimulates the immune system to produce antibodies and to "remember" the organism.

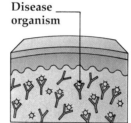

Disease organism

3 If the person is then exposed to the organism, antibodies are produced in large numbers to stop the infection.

PASSIVE IMMUNIZATION

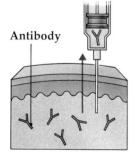

Antibody

1 Blood is taken from a number of people who have recently recovered from a particular infection. The blood contains antibodies against the disease organism.

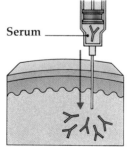

Serum

2 Serum containing the antibodies is extracted, pooled with other extracted immune serum, purified, and injected into the person being immunized.

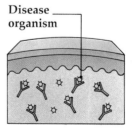

Disease organism

3 The antibodies immediately attack the disease organism if it is present, or they provide short-term protection against the organism if it enters the body.

Since the introduction of routine immunization, infectious diseases such as diphtheria and polio have become almost nonexistent. However, vaccination programs for entire populations are necessary to prevent these diseases from reappearing. If immunization against diphtheria, for example, were to stop, reintroduction of the disease from abroad could lead to a devastating epidemic with many deaths.

Most children are now immunized against the common childhood infections and against less common, but serious, diseases such as whooping cough (pertussis) and polio. Travelers to foreign countries are advised to follow specific immunization schedules so they are protected against diseases that are prevalent in those areas, especially if they are going to developing countries (see page 75). There are two types of immunization. Active immunization provides lasting immunity. Passive immunization provides immediate but short-lived immunity.

TYPES OF VACCINES

Three different forms of vaccines are used today. Inactivated vaccines are made of organisms that have been killed or inactivated by heat or chemicals; the vaccines are then purified. Vaccines of this type are used for whooping cough (pertussis), cholera, and typhoid fever.

An attenuated (weakened) vaccine consists of live organisms that have been

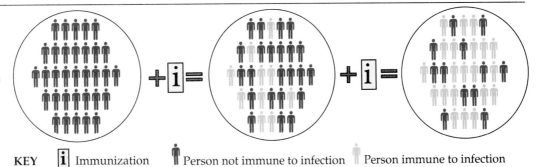

Effects of immunization
The purpose of immunization is not only to protect individuals but to gradually eliminate a disease from the world. This goal has been achieved with smallpox.

KEY **i** Immunization 🧍 Person not immune to infection 🧍 Person immune to infection

altered so that they can no longer cause infection. Although harmless, the organisms in the vaccine are able to induce immunity. Vaccines of this type are used for polio, measles, mumps, and rubella.

Some vaccines are derived from inactivated toxins produced by disease-causing organisms. Vaccines of this type are used for diseases whose symptoms are caused by the body's response to the toxins. The toxin stimulates the production of antibodies but does not produce illness. The vaccines for tetanus and diphtheria are examples of vaccines made from inactivated toxins.

Of the different types, the weakened, live vaccines generally provide the most effective, long-lasting immunity.

How vaccination works
The principle of vaccination is illustrated below with the diphtheria toxoid, an inactivated bacterial toxin that is no longer able to cause disease. After vaccination, your body's first response is to produce antibodies designed specifically to destroy the toxin. If you are subsequently exposed to diphtheria bacteria, your immune system is primed to rapidly produce antibodies to neutralize the harmful effects of the organisms.

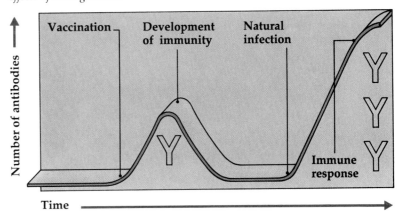

CHILDHOOD IMMUNIZATION PROGRAM	AGE	COMBINED INJECTION	ORAL
In the US, the Advisory Committee on Immunization Practices and the American Academy of Pediatrics recommend that children be vaccinated against certain infections at the ages shown at right.	2 months	Diphtheria, pertussis (whooping cough), tetanus, *Haemophilus influenzae* type b	Poliomyelitis
	4 months	Diphtheria, pertussis, tetanus, *Haemophilus influenzae* type b	Poliomyelitis
	6 months	Diphtheria, pertussis, tetanus, *Haemophilus influenzae* type b	
	15 months	Measles, mumps, rubella (German measles), *Haemophilus influenzae* type b. During outbreaks, the measles vaccine is given at 6 to 12 months with a booster at 15 months.	
	18 months	Diphtheria, pertussis, tetanus	Poliomyelitis
	4 to 6 years	Diphtheria, pertussis, tetanus	Poliomyelitis
	11 to 12 years	Measles, mumps, rubella	
	14 to 16 years	Diphtheria, tetanus. Booster needed every 10 years throughout life.	

VACCINATIONS

Most vaccinations are given by injection. A common site for injection is the outer, upper part of the arm. The polio vaccine, however, is usually given by mouth. To administer mass inoculations (for example, to military personnel), doctors often use a compressed air gun, an instrument designed to allow rapid, consecutive vaccinations of many people. Some vaccines are administered with an added substance that enhances the vaccine's effect by boosting the production of antibodies in the body. Some vaccines are now produced by genetic engineering, in which viral genetic material is incorporated into the genetic material of a living organism such as a bacterium. When the organism multiplies, the viral genes replicate at the same time, producing large quantities of viral material that can be used in vaccines. Genetically engineered vaccines, like other vaccines, trigger immune responses without causing disease.

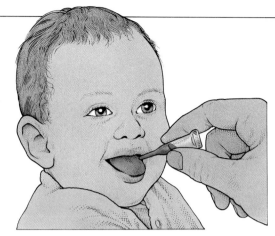

Polio vaccine
The first vaccine for polio was a killed vaccine that was given by injection into muscle. Today, doctors use a live, weakened, oral polio vaccine that is easier to administer and less expensive to produce. The polio vaccine is given in drops applied to the tongue, as shown at left.

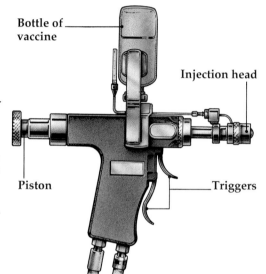

Compressed air gun
The compressed air gun uses the action of a hydraulic pump to release vaccine at such a high pressure that the liquid punctures the skin. The air gun prevents cross-infection, which can occur when disease-causing organisms are spread from one person to another with an unsterile needle. The injection can be made into a muscle or under the skin.

Bottle of vaccine

Injection head

Piston

Triggers

A GENETICALLY ENGINEERED VACCINE

A genetically engineered vaccine for hepatitis B is now available. The vaccine consists of only part of the hepatitis B virus (a protein on its surface called an antigen) but this small part can stimulate the immune system to destroy the whole virus. Many more genetically engineered vaccines will be produced in the future.

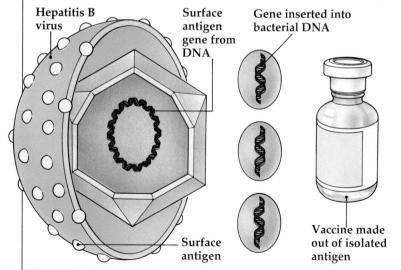

Hepatitis B virus

Surface antigen gene from DNA

Gene inserted into bacterial DNA

Surface antigen

Vaccine made out of isolated antigen

Producing the vaccine
The gene for the surface antigen is isolated from the DNA (genetic material) of the hepatitis B virus and integrated into the DNA of a bacterium. As the bacterium multiplies and produces new proteins, it also produces the viral surface antigen. This antigen is then purified for use as a vaccine.

WARNING
People with immune deficiency disorders such as AIDS, some people with cancer, and some people who take corticosteroid drugs have weakened immune systems. They risk infection if they receive a live, weakened vaccine. Anyone who has had an adverse reaction to a vaccine should not be reimmunized with that vaccine. Some vaccines should not be given to pregnant women or those planning to get pregnant within 3 months of vaccination.

RECOMMENDED VACCINATIONS FOR FOREIGN TRAVEL

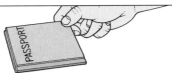

DISEASE	REASON FOR IMMUNIZATION	EFFECTIVENESS
Yellow fever	Compulsory for entry into some countries and recommended for visits to other countries in areas of Africa and South America.	Nearly 100 percent for at least 10 years.
Cholera	Sometimes compulsory for entry into countries in Asia and Africa and recommended for others.	Moderate protection for 6 months. Other precautions are necessary in areas with cholera.
Typhoid fever	Recommended everywhere outside of the US, Canada, Europe, Australia, and New Zealand.	Moderate protection for approximately 5 years. Booster is needed after this time.
Tetanus	Recommended for anyone who has not had a childhood vaccination and for those who have not had a booster within the last 10 years.	Highly effective. Booster needed every 10 years.
Polio	Recommended for anyone who has not had a childhood vaccination.	Highly effective.
Hepatitis A	Recommended for travel to any country where standards of hygiene are low and sanitation is poor.	Moderate protection for up to 3 months. Booster needed every 5 months during prolonged travel or residency.
Measles	Recommended for anyone who has not had a childhood vaccination or who has not had measles.	Effective protection previously thought to last a lifetime. Recent outbreaks have led to new recommendations.
Diphtheria	Recommended for anyone who has not had a childhood vaccination.	Highly effective. Booster needed every 10 years.
Hepatitis B Rabies Meningitis	Recommended for people at risk.	All highly effective.

ASK YOUR DOCTOR
VACCINATIONS

Q Is it true that there is a new vaccine to prevent a common cause of pneumonia and meningitis in children? When should my baby be vaccinated?

A Yes. The FDA has approved the use of two new vaccines for *Haemophilus influenzae* type b (Hib) infections in infants. The death rate from Hib infections is about 5 percent despite the availability of effective treatment. Nearly one third of the survivors have permanent brain damage. Because of the severity of this infection, vaccination is now recommended for infants at 2, 4, and 6 months, with a follow-up booster vaccination at 15 months.

Q After my last typhoid vaccination, I felt sick and my arm hurt for about 24 hours. Was this an allergic reaction?

A No. It is normal to experience pain and redness at the site of the injection. Some people also have a headache, mild fever, or tenderness in the lymph glands under their arms, or feel tired. But these symptoms quickly disappear.

Q I have heard that some vaccines, like the whooping cough vaccine, can have severe adverse effects such as brain damage. Is this true?

A Publicity often focuses on complications of this type. Some people have a life-threatening reaction to a particular vaccine, but this is extremely rare. Of greater concern is a recent increase in cases of whooping cough (pertussis) because frightened parents are not having their children vaccinated.

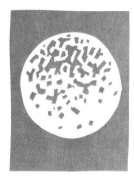

DIAGNOSING INFECTIOUS DISEASES

T O DETERMINE THE CAUSE of an infection, samples of body fluids or tissues are collected and examined under a microscope to identify disease-causing bacteria, fungi, or viruses. Sometimes viruses and other microorganisms are identified indirectly through antibody tests, which recognize antibodies that the immune system has formed in response to invasion by a particular disease organism.

For the most part, it is your body that fights infection, but it is often assisted by microbe-fighting drugs. In order for doctors to prescribe the drug that most effectively treats a particular infection, they may first need to identify the disease-causing organism. Doctors can choose from a number of tests to help them make an accurate diagnosis.

Risk factors
Certain circumstances may increase your risk of acquiring an infectious disease. Travel abroad, contact with animals, or a chronic illness such as diabetes can be risk factors. For instance, if a person who works closely with birds has a bad cough, a doctor may suspect a fungal lung infection or psittacosis (parrot fever).

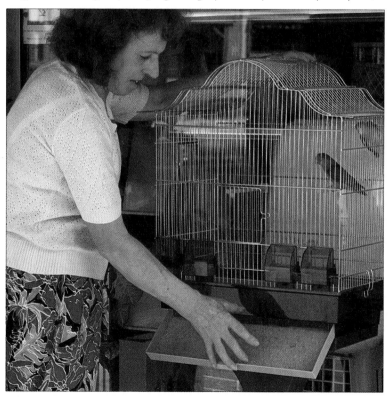

CLINICAL DIAGNOSIS

To diagnose your illness, your doctor will question you about it, examine you, and, in some cases, order tests.

Your medical history
The history of an illness is important because some disease organisms affect certain parts of the body, and pain or inflammation in a certain area may indicate a specific infection or illness. For instance, a cough usually signals a respiratory infection. Your doctor may ask you if you have recently traveled to a foreign country or if you have had contact with animals. If your doctor suspects you have a contagious infection or a sexually transmitted disease, he or she may ask you about any close physical contact you have recently had with other people, including sexual partners. Aches and pains, a headache, sore throat, and fever may indicate a generalized viral infection such as influenza.

Urine analysis
If the infection appears to be in your bladder or urethra, your doctor will ask you for a sample of urine. The sample will be sent to the laboratory to be cultured (grown under laboratory conditions) and examined.

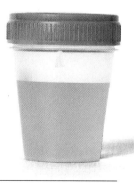

Examination

A physical examination will also help your doctor diagnose the illness. He or she will look for signs of infection such as redness, swelling, warmth, or tenderness. A heart murmur may suggest a heart valve infection; tenderness in your sides or the middle of your back may point to a kidney infection.

Tests

Your doctor may take samples from you to send to the laboratory for testing. For example, if your problem is a sore throat, your doctor will take a sample of mucus from your throat with a cotton swab. Cotton swabs are also used to take mucus from the genital area and from sores

Bacterial culture
The microbiologist shown at right is placing samples into dishes that contain agar culture media. Agar is a starchlike substance obtained from red algae (single-celled organisms that live in water). Agar is an ideal environment for multiplying bacteria because it provides them with essential nutrients.

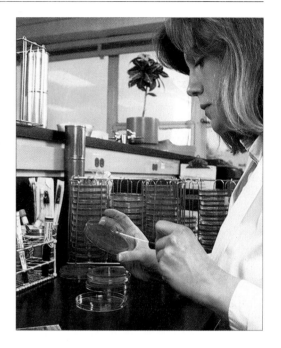

or wounds. Other samples may include blood, urine, feces, and phlegm. Your doctor may also use imaging techniques such as X-rays, ultrasound scans, and computed tomography (CT) scans to help make a diagnosis.

LABORATORY DIAGNOSIS

Microbiologists perform a wide variety of tests on body samples in the laboratory. The microbiology laboratory has incubators in which to grow bacteria, low-temperature freezers for preserving samples, and sterilizing units to decontaminate equipment. Protective hoods that cover samples guard against the escape of disease organisms. Cleanliness and protective clothing are essential to prevent contamination and the risk of infection in the laboratory.

Samples, which may be of phlegm, urine, feces, spinal fluid, or cells taken from the body, are placed on slides and examined under microscopes. Microscopes are also used to identify disease-causing organisms that have been grown on culture plates. Viruses, which are too small to be seen with an ordinary microscope, are viewed under more powerful electron microscopes.

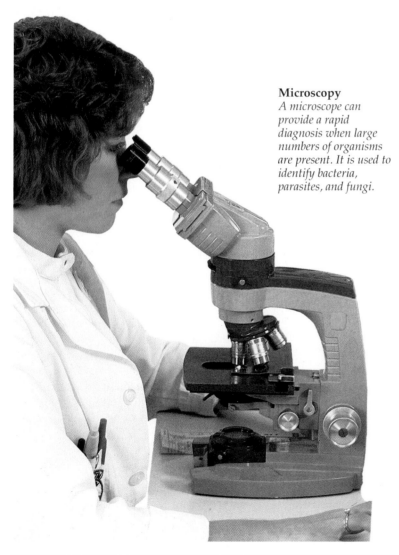

Microscopy
A microscope can provide a rapid diagnosis when large numbers of organisms are present. It is used to identify bacteria, parasites, and fungi.

SPECIAL STAINING TECHNIQUES

Because they are colorless, most organisms are difficult to see even under a microscope. Stains are dyes that help to identify disease-causing microorganisms. Gram's stain is used to distinguish between groups of bacteria, while some stains help to identify specific microbes. The Ziehl-Neelsen stain is used to help diagnose tuberculosis; a silver stain helps to diagnose fungal diseases.

GRAM'S STAIN

Preparing the slide
A sample is smeared onto a clean, glass slide and then stabilized (fixed) using heat.

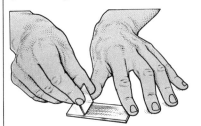

Staining
The specimen is stained with a violet dye, followed by application of iodine-based Gram's solution and then alcohol to decolorize it. The specimen is then counterstained with a red dye.

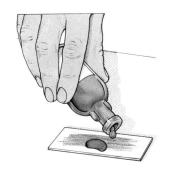

Gram-positive
Gram-positive bacteria retain the dark violet stain. They include species of streptococci and staphylococci and the organisms responsible for tetanus, diphtheria, anthrax, listeriosis, and botulism.

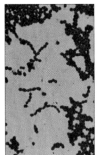

Gram-negative
Gram-negative bacteria do not retain the violet color after decolorization but take up the counterstain, appearing pink. They include various species of salmonella and the organisms that cause gonorrhea, whooping cough, and cholera.

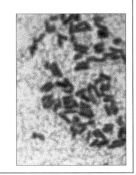

CULTURE TECHNIQUES

Germs are cultured (grown in the laboratory) to produce uncontaminated samples. Culturing is often the first step in identifying the organism that is causing your illness.

Culturing bacteria and fungi
Bacteria and fungi are grown on agar plates – plastic dishes that contain a culture medium, usually a gel called agar that is derived from algae. A culture medium provides nutrients necessary for microorganisms to grow. The sample taken from your body is smeared onto the agar plate and placed in a warm, humid environment. Each organism requires certain amounts of oxygen, carbon dioxide, and nutrients to grow. Some bloodborne bacteria grow best in agar with blood added, while some bacteria found in the intestines grow best when bile salts are added. The ideal environment of the culture medium enables the suspect disease-causing organism to multiply enough to be easily identified.

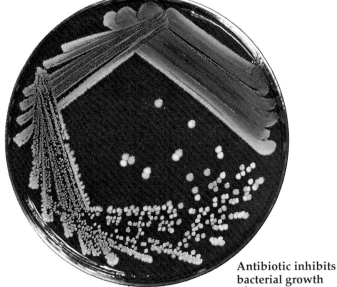

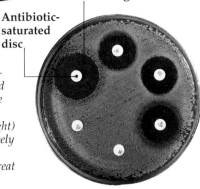

Antibiotic inhibits bacterial growth

Antibiotic-saturated disc

Antibiotic sensitivity
When the bacteria have grown into visible colonies (above), they are separated from other bacterial colonies and transferred to a new agar plate. In the new culture plate, the bacteria are exposed to a variety of antibiotics (right) to determine which ones most effectively destroy them. This information helps doctors choose the best antibiotic to treat a particular bacterial infection.

ANTIBODY TESTS

Many disease organisms stimulate the body's immune system to produce antibodies to fight them. An antibody attaches, fitting perfectly, to a specific substance located on the organism's surface. This protein substance, which triggers the immune response, is called an antigen. The immune system produces two major types of antibodies – called immunoglobulin M and immunoglobulin G – that are measured in antibody tests to determine the body's response to a specific infection. Examining a person's blood for antibodies helps identify disease-causing organisms, particularly viruses. In tests called immunoassays, antibodies are used to detect the presence of disease organisms in the blood. Some tests reverse this process, using antigens to detect the presence of antibodies that the body has produced to fight the infection. This is the type of test used to detect antibodies to HIV, the AIDS virus.

TESTS FOR VIRUSES

Because viruses cannot be cultured, indirect methods are usually used to detect them. One of these techniques examines the effect that a virus-infected sample has on cell cultures.

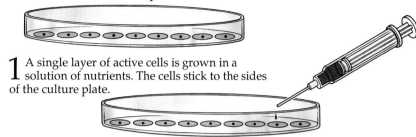

1 A single layer of active cells is grown in a solution of nutrients. The cells stick to the sides of the culture plate.

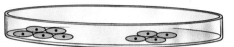

2 Blood or samples of other body fluids from the infected person are added to the plate.

3 The presence of a virus can be recognized in several ways. Here a virus causes the cultured cells to stick together (agglutination).

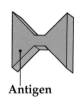

Agglutination
At left is the control slide from the virus-free culture plate. The virus-infected cells are shown clumping together in the slide at right.

ELISA TEST

The enzyme-linked immunosorbent assay (ELISA) test uses prepared antigens (fragments of disease-causing organisms) to detect antibodies produced by the body to fight a specific organism. The test is used to diagnose both viral and bacterial infections. ELISA is simple and fast; a plate of 96 tests can be read in minutes.

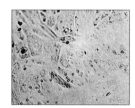

Antigen

1 Copies of a known antigen are attached to the surface of a special plastic plate.

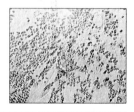

Antibody

2 If specific antibodies are present in the blood that has been added to the plate, they will bind to the antigens. Material that has not bound to the antigens is removed.

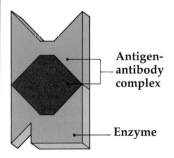

Antigen-antibody complex

Enzyme

3 A specific enzyme that will bind to the antigen-antibody complex is added. The plate is washed to remove any enzyme that has not attached.

4 A chemical that changes color when it reacts with the enzyme is added to the plate.

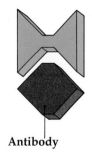

Chemical

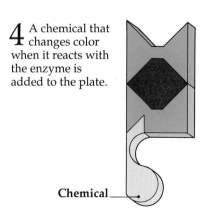

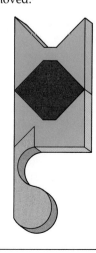

5 After a set time, the reaction is stopped and the results are determined using a spectrophotometer. This instrument uses light to estimate the level of antibodies present in the blood. The intensity of the color of the chemical is proportional to the number of antibodies present in the blood.

CHAPTER FOUR

THE RANGE OF INFECTIONS

INTRODUCTION

COLDS, INFLUENZA, AND SORE THROATS

CHILDHOOD INFECTIONS

BRAIN INFECTIONS

EYE AND EAR INFECTIONS

LUNG AND HEART INFECTIONS

DIGESTIVE TRACT INFECTIONS

VIRAL HEPATITIS

SKIN INFECTIONS AND INFESTATIONS

URINARY TRACT INFECTIONS

SEXUALLY TRANSMITTED DISEASES

Most of the epidemics that have killed large numbers of people throughout history have been caused by infectious diseases – including smallpox, plague, typhus, and yellow fever – that affect the whole body. Modern medicine has brought most of these illnesses under control. However, a few, including measles and (in tropical countries) malaria, are still widespread. Most infections today affect only one organ or tract inside the body. The most frequent so-called local infections – the common cold, tonsillitis, and sinusitis – occur in the upper respiratory tract. Other common infections affect the digestive tract, where they can cause diarrhea. The lungs, reproductive and urinary tracts, eyes, and ears are also frequent sites of infection.

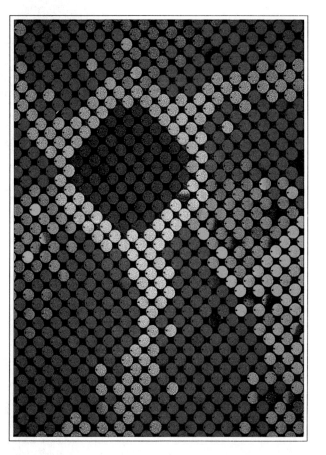

A local infection such as a boil or an inflamed eye or ear may cause severe damage to the affected organ, but the disease organisms rarely spread. While local infections are usually caused by bacteria, viral infections are sometimes localized as well. Viral conjunctivitis, for example, affects only the eye. Most localized bacterial infections, however, have the potential to spread throughout the body, causing blood poisoning that can be fatal. Viral illnesses with predominantly localized symptoms may also have phases in which the viruses are traveling through the bloodstream. Local infections can cause serious illness if they affect vital organs such as the brain, heart, or liver, or if they produce particularly damaging effects. In a person with cholera, for instance, although the bacteria remain in the intestines and do not penetrate the intestinal lining, they cause a devastating loss of fluid that can be fatal within a few hours.

Most viral and bacterial illnesses are acute (short and severe); the person either makes a full recovery from the infection within about a week or dies. Some infections can become chronic, causing progressively more severe damage. Approximately 10 to 15 percent of cases of viral hepatitis type B become chronic; slightly higher percentages of tuberculosis and untreated syphilis become chronic. Occasionally, local infections such as athletes' foot and fungal infections of the nails become chronic.

The body's immune system is more successful at fighting bacterial and viral infections than it is at eliminating parasites. Surface parasites (such as lice) that infest the skin and intestinal parasites (such as worms) may persist for years, or even a lifetime. However, most infestations and infections can be controlled or eliminated by drugs.

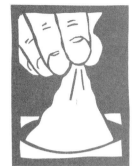

COLDS, INFLUENZA, AND SORE THROATS

People with respiratory tract infections account for nearly one out of every four visits to the doctor in the US. These common infections are usually accompanied by a sore throat, runny nose, cough, and fever, but some of them can be more serious and produce severe, debilitating illness.

Respiratory tract infections account for one third of all the time missed from work in the US. They strike children an average of six times every year. They are usually acquired when a person has close contact with an infected person or inhales or ingests germs that have been sneezed or coughed into the air.

UPPER RESPIRATORY TRACT INFECTIONS

Upper respiratory tract infections are infections of the nose, nasal sinuses, pharynx, and larynx. Viruses cause most of these illnesses, which are characterized by inflammation of the mucous membranes and underlying tissues of the affected areas. Bacterial infections are more serious and usually occur as secondary infections; that is, they result from or follow another illness. Because of the large number of different viruses and bacteria that can cause upper respiratory tract infections, it is impossible for you to become immune to all of them. Most respiratory infections are treated with painkillers only, but infections caused by bacteria, or complicated later by bacteria, are treated with antibiotics.

Sinuses

Pharynx

Tonsils

Vocal cords

Larynx

Laryngitis
Laryngitis (inflammation of the vocal cords) usually causes hoarseness, a sore throat, and loss of voice.

Tonsillitis
Tonsillitis (inflammation of the tonsils) occurs most often in children between the ages of 2 and 9. Symptoms include a sore throat, difficulty swallowing, fever, headache, earache, pus on the tonsils, and swollen lymph glands in the neck.

Pharyngitis
Pharyngitis (inflammation of the pharynx, or throat) causes a sore throat, difficulty swallowing, fever, earache, and swollen lymph nodes in the neck. The fever may be very high (particularly in children) and the soft palate and larynx may swell. If breathing becomes difficult, seek medical attention immediately.

Sinusitis
Sinusitis (inflammation of the membranes that line the cavities of the bones surrounding the nose) is often caused by a bacterial infection that develops as a complication of a viral infection. Symptoms include pain, fever, a stuffy nose, headache, and loss of the sense of smell. Sometimes pus accumulates.

COLDS AND INFLUENZA

Many people think they have the flu (influenza) when, in fact, they have a common cold. Both illnesses are caused by viruses and share many symptoms, but influenza occurs far less frequently (except during epidemics), the symptoms are more severe, and the complications are potentially much more dangerous. The common cold is an infection of the upper respiratory tract, while influenza usually affects the smaller airways in the lungs and is therefore called a lower respiratory tract infection. Pneumonia also affects the lower respiratory tract.

Cold viruses
Nearly 200 different viruses can give you a common cold. You can acquire any of these viruses in infected droplets from someone who is sneezing or coughing. Colds most often affect school children and young adults. They are usually caused by viruses called rhinoviruses (above right, magnified 11,000 times), which multiply in the cells that line the nose and are shed mainly from the nose. Viruses called coronaviruses (right, magnified 44,000 times) are the second most common cause of colds.

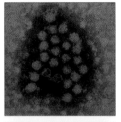
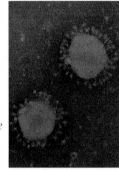

Prevalence of the common cold
This mild illness is the most common respiratory tract infection. Children can have as many as 10 colds a year because they are continually exposed to viruses to which they have not yet developed immunity. Because adults have developed immunity to many cold viruses over the years, they have fewer infections. Colds are more frequent in the winter months because people spend more time crowded together indoors where viruses can spread easily.

Symptoms of the common cold
The main symptoms of a cold – sneezing and a runny nose – are familiar to us all. Swelling of the tissue inside the nose leads to a clear, watery discharge that often thickens and turns yellow or green. Other symptoms include fever, sore throat, cough, or watery eyes. Because colds are caused by viruses, antibiotics are not effective in treating them. Your immune system can usually conquer a cold within a week, but if your cold lasts longer, or spreads beyond the nose and throat, consult your doctor.

Areas of swollen tissue

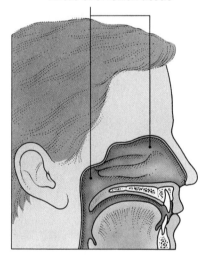

Influenza virus
Influenza is caused by viruses of the orthomyxovirus family (such as the one shown at right, magni-

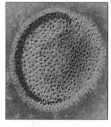

fied 300,000 times) that target the cells lining the respiratory tract. You can acquire influenza viruses from infected droplets coughed or sneezed into the air. Every few years, a new strain of influenza virus – to which most people are not immune – emerges and causes an epidemic. Epidemics vary in severity, depending on the characteristics of the specific strain of the virus.

Symptoms of influenza
Influenza is a severe illness that causes a cough, chills, fever, headache, muscle aches, weakness, and loss of appetite. These symptoms may be accompanied by a sore throat and a runny nose. Symptoms usually subside in a few days but respiratory symptoms persist, leaving you feeling weak. Influenza is life-threatening to the elderly and the very young, to people with lung and heart disease, and to people with a weakened immune system.

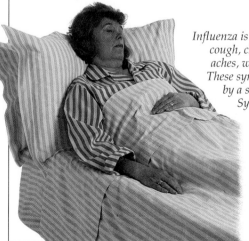

Body areas affected by influenza
Although they spread throughout the body to produce generalized symptoms, influenza viruses prefer to invade the trachea, bronchi, and lungs. Bacterial infections that occur as complications of influenza are common in the elderly and people with lung or heart disease. These bacterial infections can cause bronchitis and pneumonia, which can be life-threatening.

Trachea

Bronchi

Lungs

Influenza antigens
The outer coat of the influenza virus contains two different types of projections (surface antigens).

TYPES OF INFLUENZA

There are three different types of influenza virus – A, B, and C. Influenza spreads rapidly and tends to occur either in regional outbreaks (epidemics) or worldwide outbreaks (pandemics). Infection with any strain of influenza virus leads to immunity to that strain. However, the A and B viruses can change their structures periodically. These alterations prevent your immune system from recognizing the virus. Antibodies formed to fight the previous strain of the virus will be ineffective against the new one. For this reason, you can become sick with influenza types A and B more than once during your lifetime.

ANTIGENIC SHIFT AND ANTIGENIC DRIFT

The influenza A virus is associated with the most serious epidemics. The virus has altered its structure many times. These changes occur in the surface antigens, the triggers of the immune response. This major alteration of the virus, called antigenic shift, has led to several pandemics. In addition, both influenza A and B viruses can undergo antigenic drift, in which relatively minor changes in their surface structures occur. These minor changes do not usually lead to pandemics, but can weaken the im-

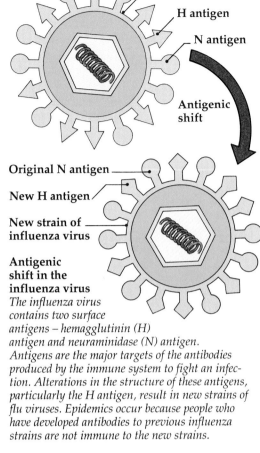

Influenza virus
H antigen
N antigen
Antigenic shift

Original N antigen
New H antigen
New strain of influenza virus

Antigenic shift in the influenza virus
The influenza virus contains two surface antigens – hemagglutinin (H) antigen and neuraminidase (N) antigen. Antigens are the major targets of the antibodies produced by the immune system to fight an infection. Alterations in the structure of these antigens, particularly the H antigen, result in new strains of flu viruses. Epidemics occur because people who have developed antibodies to previous influenza strains are not immune to the new strains.

munity that exists in populations enough to cause epidemics. Influenza B infections are generally milder than those caused by the A virus. Type C viruses cannot change their structure, so, once you have been infected by a type C virus, you acquire long-lasting immunity to it. The influenza C virus usually causes a mild illness that is indistinguishable from a common cold.

In 1978, a pandemic of influenza called the Russian flu was caused by a strain of influenza A virus identical to one that had caused an epidemic in 1950. This recurrence suggested that the virus had remained in its original form for 28 years. The pandemic mostly affected people under the age of 25, indicating that those who had been exposed to the virus in 1950 had developed immunity. Doctors realized that immunity acquired from exposure to a particular strain of influenza virus could last more than 20 years.

Death rates and influenza epidemics
The graph here shows periods since 1915 when there have been large numbers of deaths – more deaths than expected – in the US. These periods closely correlate with influenza epidemics. As can be seen, by far the most severe influenza outbreak occurred in 1918-1919; worldwide, the pandemic killed an estimated 20 million people.

Excess annual death rate per 100,000 people

5,000

1,500

1,000

500
400
300
200
100
0

1915 '20 '25 '30 '35 '40 '45 '50 '55 '60 '65 '70 '75 '80 '85 '90
Year

TREATMENTS FOR COLDS AND INFLUENZA

There is no cure for the common cold or for influenza. Most doctors recommend only the use of acetaminophen or aspirin to relieve the discomfort of a sore throat or headache or to reduce a fever. Children or adolescents with influenza or a fever should not be given aspirin because of its association with Reye's syndrome, a potentially life-threatening disorder. Antibiotics are used for colds and flu only if a bacterial infection has developed as a complication of the viral infection. Influenza infections in older people or those who have heart or lung disease or weakened immune systems may be treated with amantadine, an antiviral drug. If started very early in the course of the illness, amantadine may reduce the severity of influenza.

There is no vaccine to prevent colds, but there is a vaccine that is 80 percent effective against influenza. However, flu shots must be repeated yearly because the vaccine provides only short-lived immunity. Annual shots are recommended for people over 65 and others who are susceptible to infection or at risk from complications of influenza.

SELF-HELP FOR INFLUENZA

Although you cannot cure a case of influenza, there are several steps you can take to reduce the discomfort and speed your recovery.

◆ Get plenty of bed rest in a well-ventilated but warm room.

◆ Drink lots of fluids – at least 8 glasses per day.

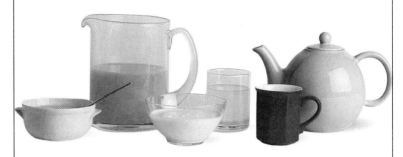

◆ Take aspirin or acetaminophen to relieve your symptoms and reduce a high fever. Children should be given only acetaminophen.

◆ Gargle with warm salt water to relieve a sore throat.

◆ If you have a high temperature, sponge yourself with lukewarm water or rubbing alcohol.

◆ Maintain a healthy diet (eat soft foods if your throat is sore).

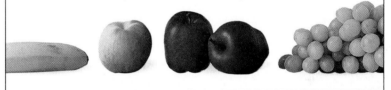

HOW CAN YOU REDUCE YOUR RISK OF A COLD?

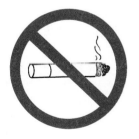

◆ Avoid close contact with anyone who has a cold.

◆ Avoid crowds.

◆ Quit smoking; smoking may reduce the efficiency of your immune system.

◆ Avoid alcohol; alcohol may reduce the efficiency of your immune system.

◆ Get enough sleep.

◆ Eat a healthy diet containing lots of fruits and vegetables.

◆ Do not share silverware or dishes at a meal.

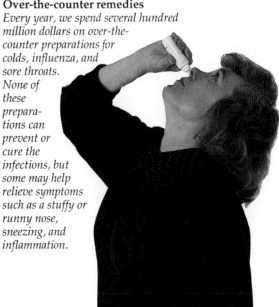

Over-the-counter remedies
Every year, we spend several hundred million dollars on over-the-counter preparations for colds, influenza, and sore throats. None of these preparations can prevent or cure the infections, but some may help relieve symptoms such as a stuffy or runny nose, sneezing, and inflammation.

INFECTIOUS MONONUCLEOSIS

Infectious mononucleosis is an acute viral infection that is also called glandular fever, mono, and kissing disease. Most infections do not produce any symptoms. Of those people who do have symptoms, 70 to 80 percent are between the ages of 15 and 30. Epidemics of infectious mononucleosis do not occur, but clustering of cases has been reported on college campuses and in military establishments. Most people recover from mononucleosis on their own. The only treatment recommended is the use of painkillers to relieve symptoms such as a fever and sore throat.

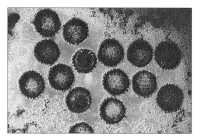

Epstein-Barr virus
More than 90 percent of all mononucleosis cases are caused by the Epstein-Barr virus (above, magnified 71,000 times), which is a member of the herpesvirus family. Most of the remaining cases are caused by cytomegalovirus, another herpesvirus. It may be 2 to 7 weeks after exposure to the virus before symptoms develop. Like all herpesviruses, Epstein-Barr virus remains in the body after infection. But unlike other herpesviruses, the virus does not appear to cause recurrent illnesses.

Symptoms of mononucleosis
The main symptoms of mononucleosis are fever, headache, a very sore throat, and swelling of the lymph glands in the neck, armpits, and groin. Tonsillitis (right), difficulty swallowing, and bleeding gums may accompany these symptoms. The spleen, which is part of the immune system, is enlarged in half the cases. The test that is used to diagnose mononucleosis identifies specific antibodies in the blood that the body has produced to fight the virus.

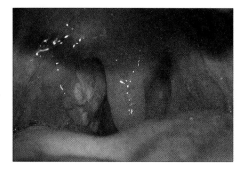

Complications
Mononucleosis may be more severe in people over the age of 30. Rare complications (including airway obstruction and inflammation of the heart) are usually treated with corticosteroid drugs. About 25 percent of people with mononucleosis develop a throat infection caused by streptococcal bacteria. The antibiotics penicillin and erythromycin are used to treat secondary infections. Some antibiotics, such as ampicillin, produce an obvious rash (left) in people who have mononucleosis.

Treatment and recovery
Treatment for mononucleosis usually consists of rest, drinking plenty of fluids, and eating a balanced diet. Aspirin or, for children, acetaminophen can help relieve symptoms. Because your spleen may become enlarged by the infection and thus susceptible to rupture, doctors recommend that you avoid strenuous exercise, particularly contact sports, for about 3 months. You may also be fatigued.

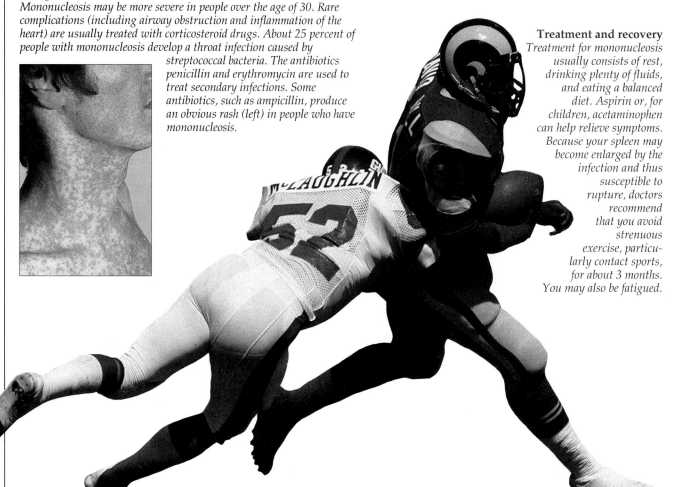

MONITOR YOUR SYMPTOMS
SORE THROAT

Most people occasionally suffer from a painful, rough, or raw feeling in their throat. Sore throats are most commonly the result of a minor infection or local irritation. A sore throat usually disappears in a few days with no treatment. However, in some cases, medical advice and treatment are necessary.

BEGIN HERE

Is your temperature 100°F (38°C) or higher?

YES

A viral infection can cause a sore throat, fever, and other symptoms.
Do you have one or more of the following?

◆ *Headache*
◆ *Cough*
◆ *Aches and pains*

NO

NO   YES

Do you have swelling and tenderness in your neck?

YES

Do you have a swollen or tender area between the angle of your jaw and ear?

NO

YES

NO

Mumps, a viral infection that affects the glands, may be causing your symptoms.

Action Consult your doctor. He or she will probably advise you to stay in bed and take aspirin or acetaminophen. In some cases, your doctor may prescribe anti-inflammatory drugs to relieve the painful swelling.

A viral infection may be the cause of your symptoms.

Action Stay in bed and, if you are an adult, take aspirin or acetaminophen. Children should have an aspirin substitute such as acetaminophen. If you do not feel better within 48 hours, see your doctor.

Pharyngitis or tonsillitis, viral or bacterial infections of the throat or tonsils, may be causing your symptoms.

Action Drink plenty of liquids and avoid solid food. Do not drink alcohol or smoke. Gargling with salt water may help. Consult your doctor if symptoms persist for more than 48 hours.

Do you have a stuffy or runny nose and/or have you been sneezing?

NO

YES

The common cold, a viral infection of the nasal passages, is probably the cause of your sore throat.

Action Keep warm, drink plenty of fluids (such as fruit juices), and take aspirin or acetaminophen. If you are prone to ear infections or bronchitis, or if you do not feel better after a week, consult your doctor.

YES

Smoking or drinking heavily can cause a sore throat.
Have you been smoking or drinking heavily or have you been in a smoky environment?

NO

Inflammation provoked by excessive smoke or alcohol has probably caused your throat to feel sore.

Action Do not smoke or drink alcohol. Restrict your diet to fluids as much as possible. Taking aspirin or acetaminophen may relieve your discomfort. Consult your doctor if your throat feels no better within 48 hours.

Are you hoarse or have you lost your voice?

YES

NO

Action Consult your doctor if you cannot make a diagnosis from this chart and your sore throat persists for more than 48 hours.

Laryngitis, inflammation of the vocal cords, is probably the cause of your symptoms.

Action Rest your voice as much as possible, drink plenty of fluids, and take aspirin or acetaminophen. If hoarseness or loss of voice persists for more than a week or recurs, consult your doctor.

87

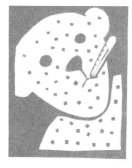

CHILDHOOD INFECTIONS

MOST CHILDHOOD ILLNESSES are caused by infections. The most common childhood infections affect the breathing passages, resulting in minor coughs, colds, and sore throats. As a child grows up, his or her immune system is continually encountering, fighting, and developing resistance to new disease organisms. By adulthood, the immune system has built up effective resistance to a wide range of infectious diseases.

Children are prone to a variety of infections, such as chickenpox, that can be recognized by characteristic symptoms and signs. However, children often have illnesses with only vague symptoms, such as a mild fever, headache, or increased irritability. Many of these illnesses are probably unidentified viral infections. The frequency of these infections diminishes as children get older.

INFECTIONS IN NEWBORNS

Newborns are susceptible to infection because their immune systems are not fully developed. Babies may contract infections either in the uterus or during passage through the birth canal. They may also acquire infections soon after birth. Most of these early infections are not serious. However, premature babies, whose immune systems are less developed than those of full-term babies, are at increased risk.

Serious infections
Although uncommon, newborns sometimes get life-threatening infections such as bacteremia (bacterial infection of blood), meningitis (inflammation of the membranes covering the brain), and pneumonia.

Eye infections cause formation of mucus and pus that can make the eyes sticky.

Thrush is a fungal (yeast) infection usually found in the mouth.

Gastrointestinal infections, such as gastroenteritis, can cause vomiting and diarrhea.

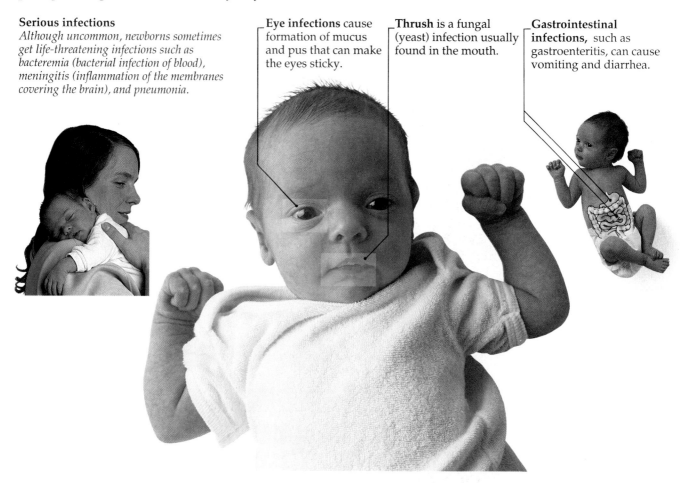

CHILDHOOD INFECTIONS

There are several infections that most children get. These infections follow consistent patterns and are easy to recognize. Usually the sick child can be cared for at home. Of the childhood infections discussed here, immunization is available only for whooping cough (pertussis). The incubation period of an illness is the time between exposure to the disease organism and the development of symptoms.

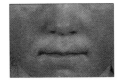

Fifth disease
Incubation period: 14 to 17 days
Fifth disease is a mild illness that often starts with a rash on the cheeks. The rash, which spreads in a lacy pattern over the arms and legs, usually disappears within 7 to 10 days. Few other symptoms are associated with the infection.

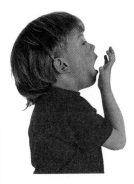

Respiratory infections
Incubation period: variable
Respiratory tract infections are the most common childhood illness. Croup, an inflammation of the breathing passages, causes children to "crow" when they breathe. Bronchiolitis, an inflammation of the small bronchi, usually affects infants that are about 4 months old. Pneumonia and bronchitis can affect adults as well as children.

Whooping cough
Incubation period: 8 to 14 days
A child with whooping cough (pertussis) becomes sick with a fever, runny nose, and cough. The "whoop" occurs when the child gasps for air. During coughing spasms, the child may turn blue and vomit. The cough usually subsides after 4 weeks; taking antibiotic drugs can shorten the illness.

Chickenpox
Incubation period: 2 to 3 weeks
The rash of chickenpox first appears on the trunk; it covers the body and sometimes the inside of the mouth. The blistering rash crusts over in a few days. The child may feel sick and have a fever until the rash fades.

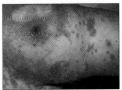

Roseola infantum
Incubation period: 7 to 14 days
Roseola infantum primarily affects children younger than 2. The infection begins with a high fever. After 3 or 4 days, the child's temperature drops and a rash (left) appears. Children usually recover from roseola within a day or two.

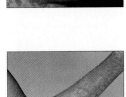

Scarlet fever
Incubation period: 2 to 6 days
This bacterial infection – which is uncommon today – begins with a fever, a headache, and a rash of fine, bright red spots. The tongue becomes inflamed and the skin on the feet, hands, and arms (left) peels. Taking penicillin may prevent the development of rheumatic fever.

Gastroenteritis
Incubation period: variable
Gastroenteritis (inflammation of the stomach and intestines) causes vomiting and diarrhea. Many types of viruses and bacteria can cause it. Although attacks are usually mild, the vomiting and diarrhea may cause dehydration, which is especially dangerous in infants.

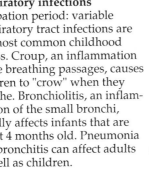

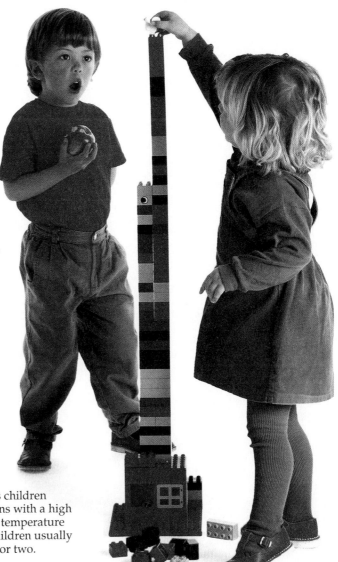

MEASLES, MUMPS, AND RUBELLA

Measles, mumps, and rubella (German measles) are viral infections that were once very common. Because of routine immunization, mumps and rubella have become rare in the US, but a recent increase in measles infections has resulted in new recommendations for measles vaccinations.

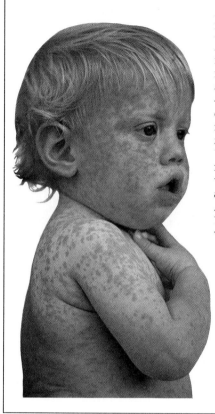

Measles
Incubation period: about 10 days
A child with measles has a fever, red eyes, a cough, and a runny nose. Tiny white spots may appear in the mouth. Within 3 or 4 days a blotchy rash develops, covering the whole body. The rash fades after 3 days. Immunization is now recommended at 15 months (in a combined measles, mumps, and rubella vaccine) or at 6 to 12 months in areas with increased incidence. A booster vaccination is given at 11 or 12 years. The follow-up vaccination is now required because infection has been occurring in teenagers who were immunized in infancy. People born after 1957 and vaccinated before 1980 should ask their doctors if they should be revaccinated. Measles can have a number of serious complications, including middle-ear infections, pneumonia, and encephalitis (inflammation of the brain).

Rubella (German measles)
Incubation period: 2 to 3 weeks
Rubella is a mild illness that frequently goes unnoticed. A rash appears, primarily on the trunk. If a woman contracts rubella during the early months of pregnancy, the disease can have devastating effects on the fetus. An infected baby may be born deaf, blind, or with heart disease.

Mumps
Incubation period: about 3 weeks
A child with mumps has a fever and may have an earache and difficulty swallowing. One or both parotid glands (the salivary glands below and in front of the ears at the angles of the jaw) become swollen and tender. Mumps sometimes causes meningitis (inflammation of the membranes that cover the brain).

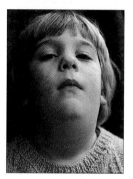

A child with mumps
The child at left has swollen parotid glands caused by mumps. In males after puberty, mumps can lead to a painful inflammation of one or both testicles.

SCHOOLS AND INFECTION

Infections spread rapidly from child to child, particularly in day-care centers and schools, where children come into close contact with each other. Preventing the spread of infection is difficult because children seldom have symptoms early in the course of the illness when it is most contagious. The incubation time (the period between exposure and development of symptoms) differs for each infection. If the infection is recognized early, the child should be kept home from school until the contagious stage of the illness has passed. Ask your doctor for information and advice.

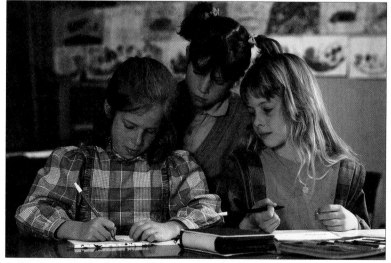

Outbreaks of infection at school
Children at school spread infections to one another easily because they are often in very close contact.

RECOGNIZING SIGNS OF AN INFECTIOUS DISEASE

Signs of illness are often harder to recognize in children than in adults. Older children may be able to describe their symptoms accurately, but irritability and crying may be the only indications of an infection in a young child. Signs may be even less obvious in newborns. Seizures are a rare complication of a quickly rising temperature in children under 2. Consult your doctor if your child has any of the following symptoms – excessive drowsiness, rapid or labored breathing, difficulty nursing or eating, recurrent diarrhea or vomiting, an unusual rash or swelling, persistent fever, or seizures.

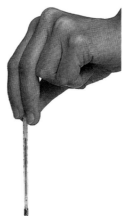

Body temperature
Normal body temperature is about 98.6°F (37°C). A high temperature in a child is not necessarily dangerous, unless it reaches 104°F (40°C) or more.

GUIDELINES FOR HOME TREATMENT

◆ Encourage your child to drink plenty of fluids to prevent dehydration and to help reduce the temperature.

◆ Give acetaminophen (available as a liquid for young children), following the dosage instructions carefully. Do not give aspirin to a child under 16.

If your child has a seizure:
◆ Lay him or her on one side. Do not put any objects or your fingers in the child's mouth. Call your doctor if your child has never had a seizure before. A seizure that lasts more than 5 minutes is an emergency.

If your child has a fever:
◆ Remove any heavy clothing and cover your child with a bed sheet.

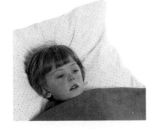

◆ Sponge your child with lukewarm water.

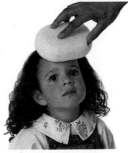

◆ If the room is hot, you may want to direct an electric fan toward your child.

ASK YOUR DOCTOR
CHILDHOOD INFECTIONS

Q My daughter had chickenpox recently and only a few spots remain on her face. Because she seems to be fine, I want to send her back to school. Should I?

A No. Chickenpox, which are like blisters at first, dry up and form scabs. A child is still very infectious until all the spots have completely dried and formed scabs.

Q My daughters, who are 9 months and 4 years old, both have whooping cough. How can I help them when they cough?

A You should cradle your baby on your lap with her head bent slightly down to keep her from swallowing vomit during a period of coughing. Your older child should be reassured and kept calm.

Q My son has chickenpox. What can I do to ease the itching and prevent him from scratching?

A Dab calamine lotion on the spots. An antihistamine can also help ease the itching. Cut your son's nails very short so that he is less able to scratch the rash. Scratching the sores increases the risk of permanent scarring.

Q When I take my child's temperature, does it make any difference if I put the thermometer under her armpit or in her mouth?

A Yes. There is a slight difference, but it is usually insignificant. When a person's temperature is taken under the arm, it is approximately 0.5°F (0.3°C) lower than when it is taken by mouth.

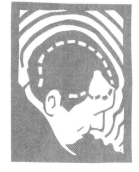

BRAIN INFECTIONS

THE BRAIN is the body's control center – any infection that involves the brain can cause devastating and often permanent harm to the body. Brain infections are rare and, since the discovery of antibiotics, permanent damage can often be avoided with early diagnosis and prompt treatment.

Infections can affect the brain itself, the membranes surrounding the brain (the meninges), or both at the same time.

Types of brain infections
Encephalitis is an infection of the brain tissue itself, while meningitis is an infection of the meninges, the membranes that surround the brain. Meningoencephalitis is an infection that affects both the brain and the meninges.

CAUSES OF BRAIN INFECTIONS

Viruses are the most common cause of encephalitis and meningitis (see left). Many different viruses – including herpesviruses, arboviruses (viruses transmitted by mosquitoes or ticks), and the mumps and measles viruses – can infect the brain and meninges. Many types of bacteria can also infect these structures. The three types of bacteria that most often cause meningitis are *Streptococcus pneumoniae*, *Neisseria meningitidis*, and *Haemophilus influenzae*. These and other bacteria sometimes cause localized brain infections called abscesses. The bacterium that causes syphilis may invade the brain if the infection has not been treated, leading to progressive brain damage and paralysis. Syphilis bacteria can also infect the spinal cord, causing pain and abnormalities of sensation.

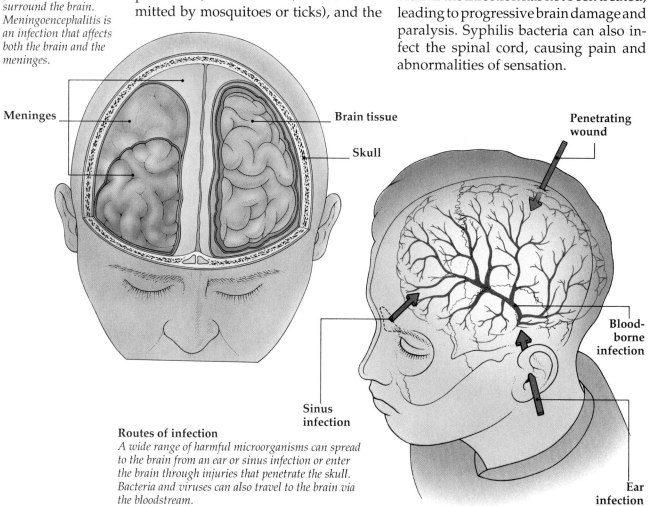

Meninges

Brain tissue

Skull

Penetrating wound

Blood-borne infection

Sinus infection

Ear infection

Routes of infection
A wide range of harmful microorganisms can spread to the brain from an ear or sinus infection or enter the brain through injuries that penetrate the skull. Bacteria and viruses can also travel to the brain via the bloodstream.

MENINGITIS

Meningitis, infection of the membranes surrounding the brain, can be fatal if it is not treated. The symptoms include a stiff neck, intolerance to light, a severe headache, and vomiting. An infected person tends to hold his or her neck rigid because any stretching of the inflamed membranes causes painful spasms.

Viral meningitis
Viral meningitis is far more common than bacterial meningitis, affecting more than 10,000 people in the US each year. Viral meningitis is usually a mild disorder but, when the virus also invades the brain itself, it can be serious. Severe cases are accompanied by headache, fever, and drowsiness that may progress to coma. Aseptic meningitis, which is usually caused by a virus, is a term also used for cases of meningitis in which the source of infection cannot be identified.

Bacterial meningitis
In adults, pneumococcal meningitis (caused by the bacterium *Streptococcus pneumoniae*) is one of the most common types of bacterial meningitis. Meningococcal meningitis (caused by the bacterium *Neisseria meningitidis*) occurs primarily in children and young adults. Small epidemics sometimes break out in institutions such as military barracks, but usually the infection occurs in isolated instances. Meningitis caused by the bacterium *Haemophilus influenzae* type b is most common in children under 6 years. For this reason, vaccinations are now required for all children.

Treatment
Treatment of meningitis involves selecting the antibiotic or antiviral drug that is most effective against the specific disease-causing organism. The sooner the infection is diagnosed and treated, the better the person's chances for recovery. One out of 3 cases of meningitis is fatal.

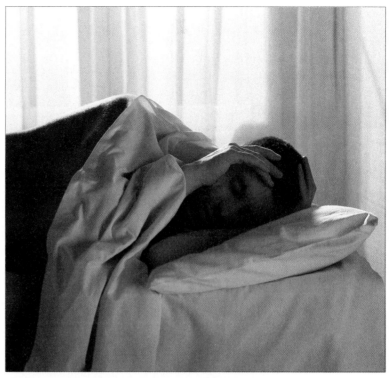

Signs and symptoms of bacterial meningitis
Fever, headache, vomiting, a stiff neck, intolerance to light, and sometimes a sore throat or a rash with red spots on the body may be symptoms of bacterial meningitis.

Diagnosis
Meningitis is diagnosed by examining a sample of fluid from the spinal canal. Fluid taken from a person with bacterial meningitis is cloudy (see left).

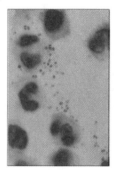

Identifying the organism
The photograph at left (magnified 1,000 times) shows the bacterium Neisseria meningitidis, *a cause of meningitis, in fluid taken from the spinal canal.*

ENCEPHALITIS

The brain is a complex organ. Infections can have varying effects on the brain. Some disease organisms concentrate on specific areas of the brain while other organisms, such as arboviruses (transmitted by mosquitoes and ticks), produce more widespread illness.

Types of encephalitis
Bacterial encephalitis often leads to the development of a collection of pus inside the brain, called a brain abscess. Signs

POLIOMYELITIS
Before widespread immunization, polio was a major cause of brain and spinal cord infections in the US. During epidemics, the death rate was 5 to 10 percent. Many people with polio lost muscular strength in their legs. Polio is still a major crippler in developing countries.

of a brain abscess include fever, headache, drowsiness, mental confusion, and seizures. Depending on the location of the abscess, other symptoms, including double vision or paralysis, may follow. If not treated, a brain abscess can be fatal.

The herpes simplex virus can cause a severe form of encephalitis, called herpes encephalitis. The onset of the illness may be sudden or it may develop over several days. Herpes encephalitis is marked by odd behavior, a state of confusion, and seizures. If untreated, the disease often progresses to coma and death.

The term arbovirus stands for arthropod-borne virus. Arthropods include mosquitoes and ticks. Arbovirus infections tend to occur in the summer and early fall when mosquitoes are biting. Symptoms include fever, headache, nausea, vomiting, lethargy, muscle aches and pains, and sensitivity to light.

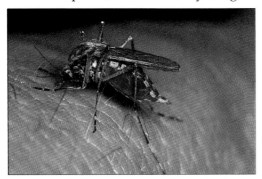

Encephalitis epidemic
The 1990 epidemic of St. Louis encephalitis, transmitted by mosquitoes, affected 27 of the 67 counties in Florida. Of the 215 cases reported, 10 were fatal.

Diagnosis and treatment
Encephalitis is usually diagnosed by laboratory tests, which may include a lumbar puncture – a procedure in which a hollow needle is inserted into the spinal canal to withdraw a sample of fluid. Bacterial encephalitis is treated with intravenous antibiotics and surgical drainage of an abscess, should one develop. There is no specific treatment for most types of viral encephalitis, but herpesvirus infections can be treated with the antiviral drug acyclovir.

RABIES

Rabies is a viral infection transmitted by the saliva of an infected animal when it bites a person or licks an open sore. Rabies viruses enter the nervous system and travel to the brain. The period between bite and appearance of symptoms may range from 14 days to 2 months or more. Once symptoms develop, rabies is fatal. An infected person becomes anxious and disoriented and has a stiff neck and seizures. The characteristic symptom of rabies is hydrophobia, which means "fear of water." Attempts to drink trigger spasms in the throat muscles that cause gagging, choking, and panic. Any person bitten by an animal should wash the area thoroughly with soap and water and seek medical advice immediately. Prompt administration of the rabies vaccine and rabies antibodies is lifesaving if given before symptoms develop.

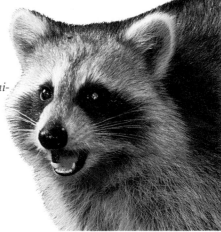

Animal carriers
Both wild and domestic animals can be infected with rabies but, in the US, skunks, raccoons, and bats are the primary carriers. Almost no reported cases of rabies are acquired from dogs in the US because they are vaccinated. However, more than half of the rabies cases among Americans result from exposure to dogs in other countries.

Rabies infection
The photograph below (magnified 55,000 times) shows the rabies virus in an animal's brain tissue.

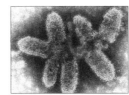

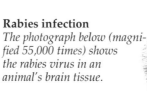

CASE HISTORY
A TROUBLING CHANGE IN BEHAVIOR

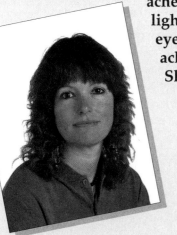

BETH HAD BEEN HAVING **repeated attacks of tonsillitis. Her health problems were beginning to affect her work. One morning, she awoke with a severe headache and noticed that the bright light in her bedroom bothered her eyes. She also had a fever and aches and pains all over her body. She decided to call her doctor.**

PERSONAL DETAILS
Name Beth Shapiro
Age 28
Occupation Fashion designer
Family Beth's mother and father are in excellent health.

MEDICAL BACKGROUND
Beth has always been healthy, although she sometimes has irritable bowel syndrome.

THE CONSULTATION
The doctor examines Beth and finds that she has a fever. He also notices that she is behaving oddly. She is not making sense and she seems disoriented. The doctor decides to send Beth to the hospital.

IN THE HOSPITAL
In the hospital, Beth is confused and inattentive. The right side of her body is weak and she behaves bizarrely – she even accuses the nurses of spying on her and trying to poison her. A few hours after admission, Beth has a seizure.

FURTHER INVESTIGATION
Beth's doctor thinks she has a type of encephalitis (an infection of the brain), but more tests need to be performed. In a procedure called a lumbar puncture, fluid is taken from Beth's spinal canal through a hollow needle. Laboratory tests show that the fluid is under abnormally high pressure and that it has a high count of both white and red blood cells. The results of an electroencephalogram (EEG) show periodic abnormal electrical discharges from Beth's brain. A magnetic resonance imaging (MRI) scan shows inflamed areas on both sides of her brain.

THE DIAGNOSIS
Based on the history of Beth's illness and the laboratory results, the doctor determines that she has HERPES ENCEPHALITIS. He explains that doctors do not know how the infection develops. The findings of the lumbar puncture, the EEG, and the MRI make him feel confident that Beth does not need to have a brain biopsy to confirm the diagnosis.

THE TREATMENT
Beth is given acyclovir intravenously. Acyclovir is a potent antiviral drug that is effective against herpesviruses. Within several days, her condition improves and after 2 weeks she is able to leave the hospital. Beth's doctor tells her she is fortunate that her illness was diagnosed and treated early enough for her to escape permanent brain damage. Her recovery is complete and she returns to work.

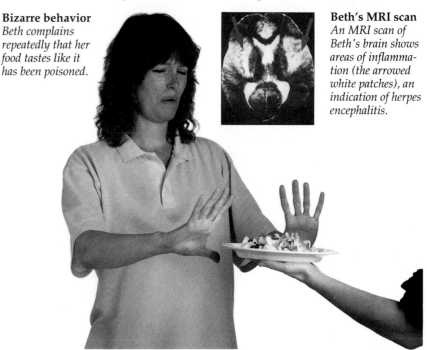

Bizarre behavior
Beth complains repeatedly that her food tastes like it has been poisoned.

Beth's MRI scan
An MRI scan of Beth's brain shows areas of inflammation (the arrowed white patches), an indication of herpes encephalitis.

EYE AND EAR INFECTIONS

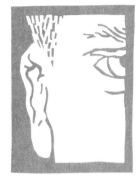

T HE EYES AND EARS are among the most common sites of infection in the body. Because infections thrive in a dark, warm, moist environment, the ear provides an ideal setting. The eyes are susceptible because of the moist, exposed, conjunctival membrane covering the white of the eye, which makes a good breeding ground for infectious organisms.

Neonatal ophthalmia
This baby has the characteristic sign of neonatal ophthalmia – a discharge of sticky pus (seen here in the left eye). Any newborn baby with sticky or inflamed eyes should be checked by a doctor immediately.

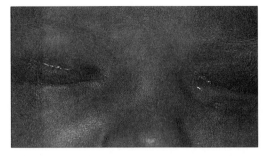

Eye infections can begin early in life and may even be acquired during birth (see illustration above and EYE INFECTION AT BIRTH below left). In babies, a discharge from the eye and tearing may mean that the tear duct has failed to open. Instead of being washed away, organisms accumulate in the upper part of the duct.

EYE INFECTION AT BIRTH

An eye infection in a newborn can cause blindness, particularly if an organism such as the bacterium that causes gonorrhea is involved. For this reason, a baby who has a discharge of pus from the eyes in the first 10 days of life should be examined by a doctor and treated promptly. To prevent these infections, most states require that medication be instilled into a baby's eyes immediately after birth to kill any organisms that may be present.

CONJUNCTIVITIS

Most eye infections involve the conjunctiva, the transparent membrane that covers the whites of the eyes and the insides of the eyelids. An inflamed conjunctiva looks red and secretes more tears and mucus than normal; the tears and mucus may combine with white blood cells that have gathered in the area, forming a heavy, cloudy or yellowish discharge. The discharge can build up during the day or night. People with conjunctivitis usually wake up in the morning with their eyelashes stuck together by dried discharge. Conjunctivitis may also be caused by an allergic reaction, but, in these cases, the discharge is clear.

Infectious conjunctivitis is most often caused by bacteria or viruses. Viral conjunctivitis, which can spread rapidly in schools and other group settings, usually clears up without treatment. Bacterial conjunctivitis requires treatment with antibiotic drops or ointment.

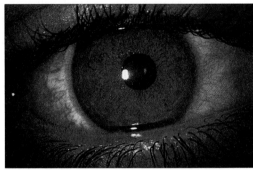

Conjunctivitis
The photograph above shows conjunctivitis caused by a chlamydial infection. Normally, the blood vessels in the conjunctiva are so fine that they are barely visible. But when the conjunctiva becomes inflamed, these tiny vessels widen and the membrane becomes noticeably red.

KERATITIS

Infection of the cornea, known as infectious keratitis, is rare compared with conjunctivitis and is a much more serious infection. Many microorganisms can cause keratitis but the herpes simplex virus is one of the most common. A herpes infection of the cornea is usually painful – a tiny ulcer that develops on the cornea often produces a feeling of grittiness in the eye that intensifies each time the person blinks. To prevent long-term damage or discomfort, infectious keratitis should be treated promptly and thoroughly with an ointment or drops containing an antiviral drug.

SITES OF EYE INFECTION

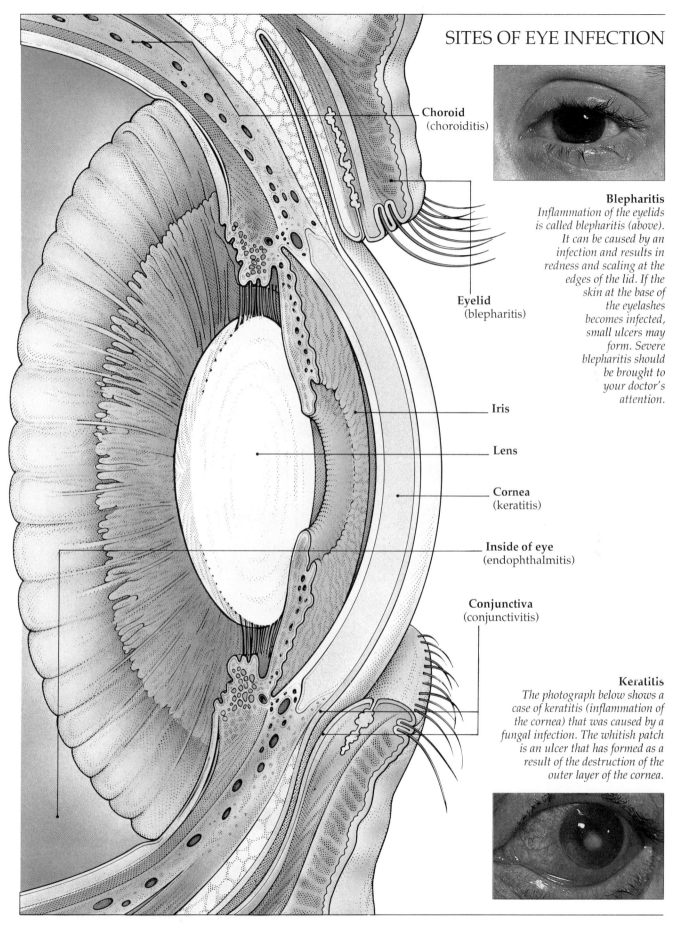

Choroid
(choroiditis)

Eyelid
(blepharitis)

Iris

Lens

Cornea
(keratitis)

Inside of eye
(endophthalmitis)

Conjunctiva
(conjunctivitis)

Blepharitis
Inflammation of the eyelids is called blepharitis (above). It can be caused by an infection and results in redness and scaling at the edges of the lid. If the skin at the base of the eyelashes becomes infected, small ulcers may form. Severe blepharitis should be brought to your doctor's attention.

Keratitis
The photograph below shows a case of keratitis (inflammation of the cornea) that was caused by a fungal infection. The whitish patch is an ulcer that has formed as a result of the destruction of the outer layer of the cornea.

OTHER EYE INFECTIONS

Endophthalmitis is an infection inside the eye that occurs after an injury that has penetrated the eye or, in rare cases, after major eye surgery. Even if this extremely serious condition is treated promptly, it is difficult to cure and removal of the eye may be necessary.

Choroiditis, an inflammation in the network of blood vessels that lines the back of the eye, may occur as a result of some infections, including tuberculosis. Corticosteroid drugs are sometimes used to treat the inflammation, and antibiotics may be used to fight the disease-causing organism.

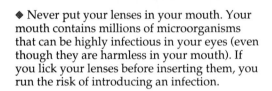

KEEPING YOUR CONTACT LENSES CLEAN

Because they come into such close and prolonged contact with the moist membranes of the eye, contact lenses are a frequent source of eye infections. It is essential to maintain a high standard of cleanliness when caring for, handling, and inserting your lenses. If you develop a serious or recurrent infection, you may not be able to continue wearing contact lenses. You may even lose your vision.

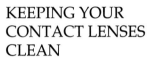

◆ Never put your lenses in your mouth. Your mouth contains millions of microorganisms that can be highly infectious in your eyes (even though they are harmless in your mouth). If you lick your lenses before inserting them, you run the risk of introducing an infection.

◆ Be meticulous about cleaning and storing your lenses. Containers can easily become contaminated and transfer germs to the lenses. Changing the soaking solution is not enough. You should sterilize the containers and lenses according to the manufacterer's instructions and replace the solution at the recommended intervals.

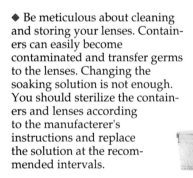

◆ Remove your contact lenses before you swim. Microorganisms, mostly bacteria, that live in lake, ocean, and unchlorinated pool water can infect your eyes.

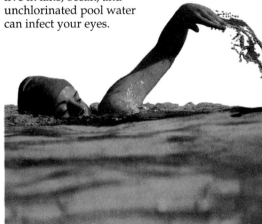

◆ Always wash your hands thoroughly before putting in or removing contact lenses. Your fingers are always contaminated with bacteria and other infectious organisms, and these organisms are easily transferred to your lenses and then to your eyes.

CASE HISTORY
PROBLEMS WITH A CONTACT LENS

SUSAN HAD WORN **soft contact lenses for 9 years with no problems, so she was surprised when her right lens began to bother her at work one day. Cleaning the lens did not help, so she decided to take her contacts out for the rest of the day. Even after the lens was out, Susan's eye still hurt considerably and began to water constantly. The next morning her eye was no better, so she went to see her doctor.**

PERSONAL DETAILS
Name Susan Ferguson
Age 27
Occupation Gym teacher
Family Both Susan's parents are healthy.

MEDICAL BACKGROUND
Susan is healthy and athletic. She swims and goes to aerobics classes regularly. Other than nearsightedness, for which she wears contact lenses, Susan has no significant medical problems.

THE CONSULTATION
Susan's doctor notices that the upper lid of her right eye is swollen and that the eye is severely inflamed. He thinks that she may have developed an allergic reaction in one eye, but he recommends that she have an ophthalmologist look at it.

THE OPHTHALMOLOGIST'S CONSULTATION
The ophthalmologist asks Susan about her experience with her contact lenses, the hours that she wears them, and her cleaning routine. She tells him that she has stopped using commercial lens solutions for storing her lenses and has been making her own saline solution with unboiled tap water. He checks Susan's vision and finds that he cannot correct the vision in her right eye to better than 20/200. With some difficulty he examines her eyes with a slit lamp, which is an illuminated microscope. He notices that the transparent membrane (conjunctiva) covering the white of her right eye is swollen and inflamed and the cornea has an irregularity at the center and an opaque ring around the edge. He takes tissue from the cornea and sends it to the laboratory for examination.

THE DIAGNOSIS
When the tissue from Susan's cornea is stained and examined under a microscope, tiny organisms are visible. The finding confirms the ophthalmologist's diagnosis that Susan has KERATITIS, an infection of the cornea. In Susan's case, the keratitis is caused by a type of ameba called *Acanthamoeba*. Susan's infection has probably occurred because of her use of the homemade, unsterile saline solution in which the amebae were later discovered.

THE TREATMENT
Susan applies antimicrobial eye drops, and the infection subsides in a few weeks. Her doctor tells her that, in many cases, this type of infection cannot be controlled with drops. Surgical removal of the infected cornea and a corneal transplant are sometimes necessary to eliminate the organisms or the scarring caused by the infection. The infection has produced a deep, dense, central, opaque area in Susan's cornea that severely reduces her vision. She finds it difficult to teach with this handicap. Susan and her doctor agree that a central corneal transplant is the best course of action.

THE OUTLOOK
The transplant is successful, and Susan's vision is restored to its previous state. Susan decides to wear glasses instead of contacts.

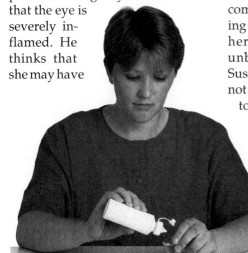

Risk of infection
Never make your own saline solution for storing your contacts. Amebae that can thrive in tap water are a cause of eye infections.

EAR INFECTIONS

Infections of the outer and middle ear can lead to two inflammatory conditions – otitis externa and otitis media.

Otitis externa

The term otitis externa is used for any inflammation of the skin of the outer ear, particularly the skin in the ear canal. This kind of inflammation, which is common, is usually caused by infections, but sometimes skin disorders such as eczema are responsible. Although a wide variety of organisms can produce outer-ear infections, the majority are caused by bacteria. Staphylococcal bacteria may infect a hair root inside the ear, forming a boil. Because the skin in the ear canal is very tight, this kind of infection can be extremely painful.

Fungal infections of the ear canal can be caused by many different fungi including *Candida albicans*, the organism that frequently causes yeast infections. Symptoms include pain and intense itching, and the skin of the ear canal may become swollen and thickened.

Treatment of outer-ear infections depends on their cause. Your doctor will probably clean out the ear canal, sometimes using a suction device, and then prescribe an antibiotic or antifungal drug.

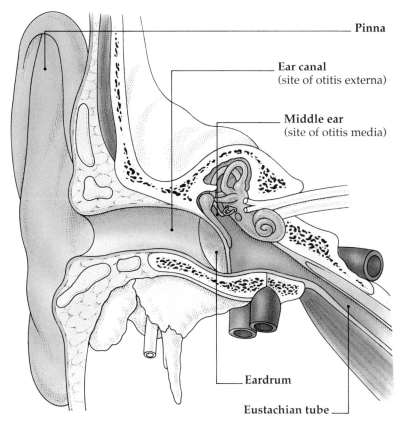

Pinna

Ear canal
(site of otitis externa)

Middle ear
(site of otitis media)

Eardrum

Eustachian tube

Ear drops
For an outer-ear infection, your doctor may prescribe ear drops containing an antibiotic or antifungal drug. Have someone put in the drops while you lie on your side. Stay lying down for a few minutes to allow the drops to penetrate the ear canal.

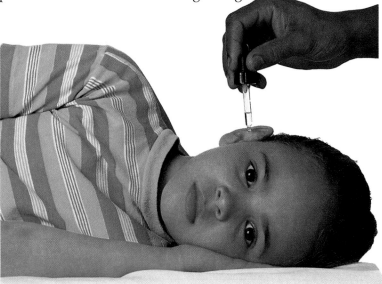

Otitis media

Otitis media is an inflammation of the middle-ear cavity and is almost always caused by infection. The infection usually spreads up to the middle ear from the nose or throat through the eustachian tube. When the tube stays open, infection is unlikely because fluid secretions drain away from the ear. However, when the tube is blocked by enlarged adenoids or by inflammation in the tube itself, an acute middle-ear infection can develop. Children are especially susceptible, probably because their eustachian tubes are short and there is

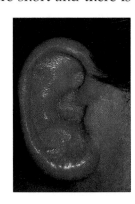

Otitis externa
Although the inflammation from an outer-ear infection is usually confined to the ear canal, some cases spread to the visible external part of the ear (the pinna), as shown at right.

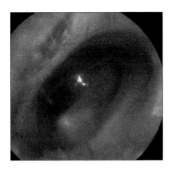

Inflamed eardrum
In acute otitis media, the eardrum reddens and bulges out, as seen here through an otoscope (an instrument used to view the inside of the ear).

not enough supportive cartilage to keep the tubes open and draining normally.

In acute otitis media, pus forms and causes the eardrum to bulge outward. The person has a severe earache, a feeling of fullness in the ear, hearing loss, ringing or buzzing in the ear (tinnitus), and fever. Treatment with oral antibiotics and analgesics (painkillers) usually clears up the infection.

Otitis media can have serious complications if the infection spreads to the mastoid bone behind the ear or from there to the brain. But if the infection is treated promptly, complications are unlikely to develop.

Middle-ear effusion

Persistent middle-ear effusion – a condition in which fluid accumulates in the middle ear – primarily affects children. It sometimes occurs as a complication of an incompletely healed middle-ear infection. A sticky fluid that accumulates in the middle ear can cause some loss of hearing. Middle-ear effusion is treated with antibiotics but, if the condition becomes chronic, surgery may be required to insert a tube to allow the ear to drain.

Helping fluid to drain
An opening is made in the eardrum and a small tube is inserted into the hole (as shown below) to allow air in and fluid to drain. Removing the adenoids may also be necessary to clear up a persistent problem.

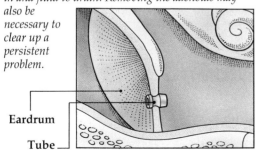

Eardrum

Tube

TAKING CARE OF YOUR EARS

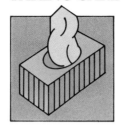

◆ Blowing your nose without pinching either nostril shut can help you avoid middle-ear infections. Holding a nostril shut when you blow raises the pressure in your nose, which can force infected mucus along the eustachian tubes into your middle ears.

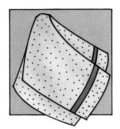

◆ Don't put anything in your ears. Infections of the outer ear can occur when the skin is scratched by items such as bobby pins, matchsticks, paper clips – or even fingernails. Gently clean the outer part of your ear with a damp washcloth to remove any dirt and obvious wax. Never use a cotton-tipped swab to clean wax out of your ears because you can easily push infected material or wax farther into the ear and damage your eardrum.

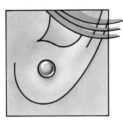

◆ When you have your ears pierced, choose a doctor or jeweler who uses disposable needles or a piercing gun that forces a sterile stud through the earlobe. Keep the wires or studs clean and handle them as little as possible. Put earrings through your ears carefully so they do not scratch the skin. Get in touch with your doctor right away if you develop an infection in your earlobes.

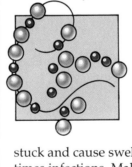

◆ Teach your children never to put objects in their ears. Items such as beads, buttons, vitamins, pebbles, and beans can get stuck and cause swelling and sometimes infections. Make sure that toys do not have small parts that might detach. Attempts to remove such objects usually push them farther into the ear, and your doctor may have to remove the object with a special instrument.

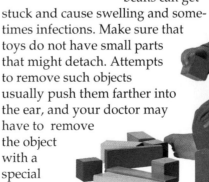

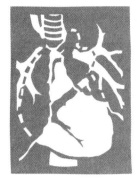

LUNG AND HEART INFECTIONS

THE AIR WE BREATHE teems with microorganisms, making it easy for us to acquire infections in our lungs and lower airways. By contrast, heart infections are rare. Although, like the lungs, the heart is located in the chest, it is isolated from the outside environment. Infectious organisms reach the heart primarily through the bloodstream.

Effects of smoking
Tobacco smoke irritates the lining of your air passages, causing them to become thickened and to secrete thick mucus. These secretions provide an opportunity for bacteria to multiply deep inside the lungs, causing recurrent infections and chronic bronchitis.

Many lung infections develop from the spread of, or from complications resulting from, infections of the upper respiratory tract – the nose, throat, and windpipe.

LUNG INFECTIONS

Common lung infections include bronchitis, bronchiolitis (inflammation of the lower airways), and many types of pneumonia. Less common lung infections include tuberculosis, lung abscesses, and pleurisy.

Bronchitis
Acute bronchitis is caused by a bacterial infection of the bronchi, the large airways to the lungs. The symptoms of acute bronchitis include coughing and coughing up infected mucus (phlegm). The infection usually clears up after treatment with antibiotics.

Chronic bronchitis is usually caused by cigarette smoking. The smoker has a chronic cough and excessive production of mucus. The most effective way to improve the condition is to quit smoking.

Pneumonia
Pneumonia is an infection in the lungs that causes inflammation and secretion of a sometimes bloody, protein-rich fluid into the air spaces of the lungs. Symptoms include a fever, cough, phlegm production, and shortness of breath. A person who has pneumonia may also have pleurisy, which is a painful inflammation of the membranes that cover the lungs and line the chest wall (see PLEURAL MEMBRANES on page 105).

Lungs of a smoker
The photograph at right shows the lungs of a person who smoked heavily for many years. The black patches are tar deposits from cigarette smoke. The arrow is pointing to a large cancerous growth.

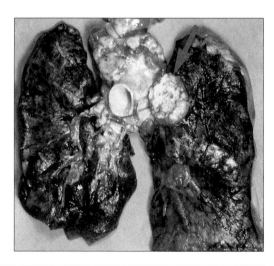

INVESTIGATING PNEUMONIA

If pneumonia is suspected, the doctor looks for characteristic signs during the physical examination and on a chest X-ray. Cultures of phlegm and blood, along with blood tests to detect antibodies, help identify the cause of the illness.

Evidence of pneumonia
The chest X-ray at right shows pneumonia in the right lung. The hazy area in the lower part of the right lung (left side of X-ray film) is swollen lung tissue filled with thick, infected secretions.

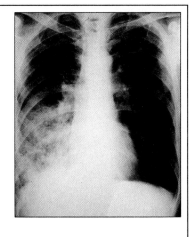

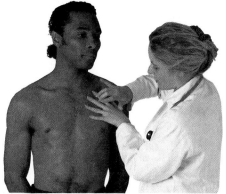

Physical examination
The doctor hears crackling sounds, called rales, coming from the lungs. Tapping the chest with the fingers produces a dull sound that indicates a buildup of fluid in the air spaces.

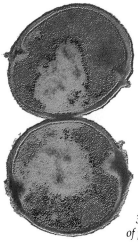

Bacterial cause of pneumonia
The bacterium Streptococcus pneumoniae *(shown in the color-enhanced photograph at left, magnified 39,000 times) is the most common cause of pneumonia in the US.*

Pneumonia is caused by many types of bacteria and viruses. Various types of fungi also sometimes cause pneumonia.

Treatment and outcome of pneumonia

People with bacterial or fungal pneumonia are treated with antibiotics or antifungal drugs. Viral pneumonia does not respond to treatment but a secondary bacterial infection that might develop would be treated with antibiotics. Secondary infections are infections that result from or follow an initial illness.

Most people recover completely from pneumonia infections. However, in someone (particularly an older person) who has a damaged lung or is ill from a debilitating disease such as cancer or AIDS, pneumonia can be fatal.

Legionnaires' disease

Legionnaires' disease, a type of pneumonia, is caused by the bacterium *Legionella pneumophila*. The organism lives in warm water and thrives in standing water in the air conditioning or plumbing systems of large buildings (see page 70). More than 1,000 cases of the disease were reported in the US in 1989. Early symptoms of legionnaires' disease include headache, muscle and stomach pain, diarrhea, and a dry cough. The disease primarily affects older people and heavy smokers and drinkers.

Lung abscess
In some cases of lung infection – particularly when treatment is delayed or the disease-causing bacteria are especially harmful – the tissue deep inside the lungs breaks down to form a pus-filled cavity, or abscess. The CT scan at right shows three abscesses (circled). The person constantly coughs up mucus that may be streaked with blood. A long-term course of antibiotics is the usual treatment. However, surgical removal of the abscess and surrounding tissue is sometimes necessary.

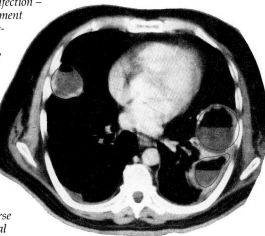

SITES OF LUNG INFECTIONS

The lungs and the branching airways that supply them (the bronchi and the bronchioles) form the lower respiratory tract. Microorganisms can cause infections at many different sites throughout these structures.

Trachea
The trachea, or windpipe, is a tube made of smooth muscle, elastic connective tissue, and fibrous cartilage tissue. The trachea connects the larynx (the voice box) to the main bronchi.

Bronchi
The primary bronchi are the two main air passages to the lungs. One bronchus supplies air to the left lung while the other supplies air to the right lung. Inside a lung, each main bronchus branches into smaller main stem and then segmental bronchi. The bronchi are the sites of infection in bronchitis.

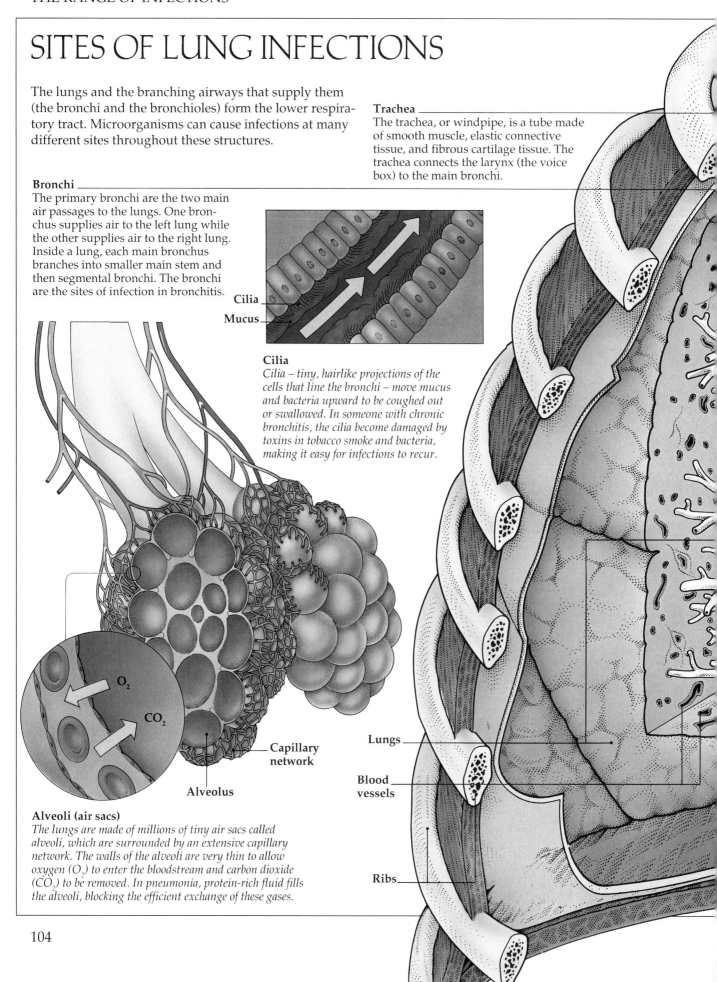

Cilia
Mucus

Cilia
Cilia – tiny, hairlike projections of the cells that line the bronchi – move mucus and bacteria upward to be coughed out or swallowed. In someone with chronic bronchitis, the cilia become damaged by toxins in tobacco smoke and bacteria, making it easy for infections to recur.

O_2

CO_2

Capillary network

Alveolus

Lungs

Blood vessels

Ribs

Alveoli (air sacs)
The lungs are made of millions of tiny air sacs called alveoli, which are surrounded by an extensive capillary network. The walls of the alveoli are very thin to allow oxygen (O_2) to enter the bloodstream and carbon dioxide (CO_2) to be removed. In pneumonia, protein-rich fluid fills the alveoli, blocking the efficient exchange of these gases.

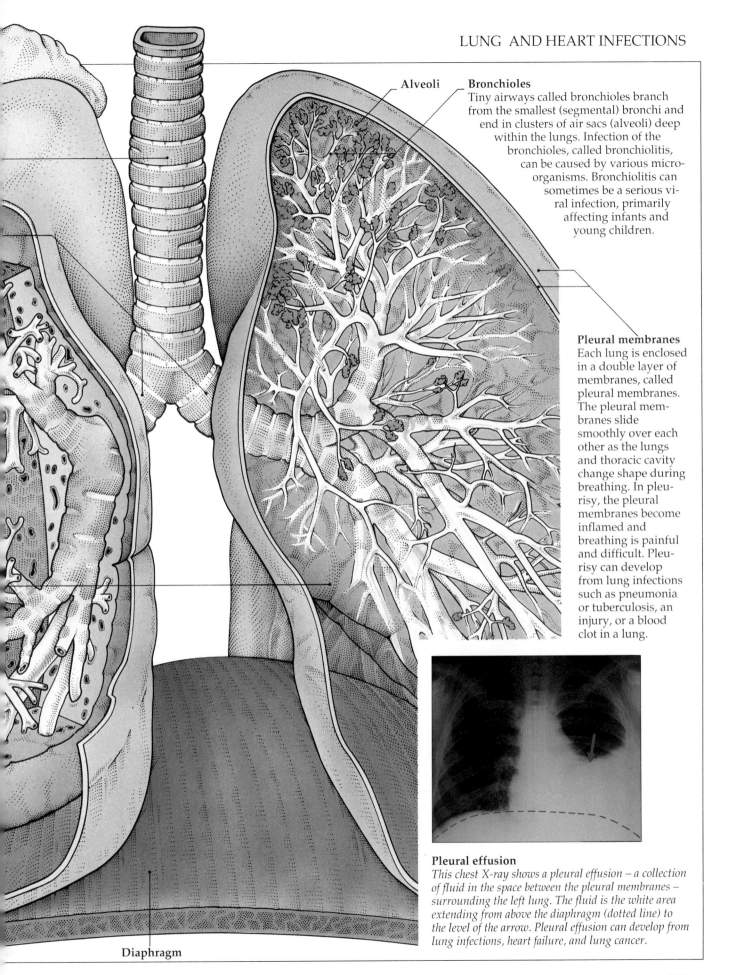

Alveoli

Bronchioles
Tiny airways called bronchioles branch from the smallest (segmental) bronchi and end in clusters of air sacs (alveoli) deep within the lungs. Infection of the bronchioles, called bronchiolitis, can be caused by various micro-organisms. Bronchiolitis can sometimes be a serious viral infection, primarily affecting infants and young children.

Pleural membranes
Each lung is enclosed in a double layer of membranes, called pleural membranes. The pleural membranes slide smoothly over each other as the lungs and thoracic cavity change shape during breathing. In pleurisy, the pleural membranes become inflamed and breathing is painful and difficult. Pleurisy can develop from lung infections such as pneumonia or tuberculosis, an injury, or a blood clot in a lung.

Pleural effusion
This chest X-ray shows a pleural effusion – a collection of fluid in the space between the pleural membranes – surrounding the left lung. The fluid is the white area extending from above the diaphragm (dotted line) to the level of the arrow. Pleural effusion can develop from lung infections, heart failure, and lung cancer.

Diaphragm

PHYSICAL OR POSTURAL THERAPY

Mucous secretions may build up in the airways connecting the trachea to the lungs of a person with a lung infection such as chronic bronchitis or an inherited lung disorder such as cystic fibrosis. Different techniques, such as those described below, may be used to try to loosen and drain fluid from the lungs to help prevent as well as treat infections.

Positions for draining lungs
By lying in different positions, a person can drain secretions from each part of the lungs. For example, the person can lean over the edge of a bed with his or her head on the floor or lie in a knee-to-chest position in bed or on the floor.

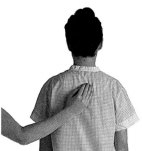

Clapping
Clapping on a person's chest with a cupped hand can help loosen sticky secretions in the lungs. Hospital personnel or a friend or family member can do the clapping.

of tuberculosis had declined steadily for many years (see below). But in some groups – such as the homeless, the undernourished, alcoholics, people with AIDS, and some immigrants – the disease is currently on the rise. People with AIDS are also susceptible to infection by *Mycobacterium avium-intracellulare*, an organism similar to the one that causes tuberculosis. However, unlike tuberculosis, the illness it causes is not transmitted from an infected person to healthy people and it is more difficult to treat.

Fungal lung infections
Fungal lung infections, which often affect people whose immune systems are impaired, can cause inflammation of the lungs. People acquire them by inhaling airborne particles contaminated with a disease-causing fungus. The most common fungal lung infections include candidiasis (a yeast infection), aspergillosis (caused by a fungus found in decaying plants), and histoplasmosis and cryptococcosis (each caused by a fungus found in bird droppings). Coccidioidomycosis (San Joaquin Valley fever) occurs only in parts of California, Arizona, and New Mexico.

Tuberculosis
Tuberculosis, which is caused by the bacterium *Mycobacterium tuberculosis*, most often affects the lungs. Early symptoms include mild fever, a slight weight loss, or a cough. Initial infection usually occurs in childhood and may go undetected. A positive skin test result or X-ray might be the only evidence of exposure. However, without effective preventive treatment, the bacteria remain in the body and may at some time become active, destroying lung tissue and blood vessels. If the infection spreads to other parts of the body, it can be life-threatening.

Tuberculosis is now a highly treatable illness. To eliminate the infection, a person takes a combination of antibiotics for at least 6 months. In the US, the incidence

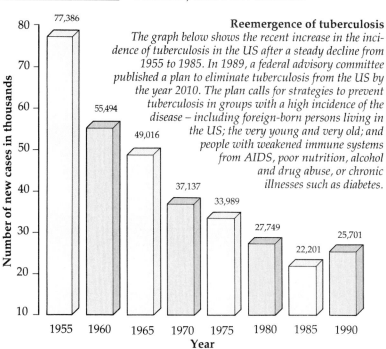

Reemergence of tuberculosis
The graph below shows the recent increase in the incidence of tuberculosis in the US after a steady decline from 1955 to 1985. In 1989, a federal advisory committee published a plan to eliminate tuberculosis from the US by the year 2010. The plan calls for strategies to prevent tuberculosis in groups with a high incidence of the disease – including foreign-born persons living in the US; the very young and very old; and people with weakened immune systems from AIDS, poor nutrition, alcohol and drug abuse, or chronic illnesses such as diabetes.

Number of new cases in thousands — Year

77,386 (1955); 55,494 (1960); 49,016 (1965); 37,137 (1970); 33,989 (1975); 27,749 (1980); 22,201 (1985); 25,701 (1990)

CASE HISTORY
A FLULIKE ILLNESS

DAVID IS A MIDDLE MANAGER at a large trade association. He developed what seemed to be a mild case of influenza with a cough and fever. Assuming his illness would clear up quickly, David did not stay home from work. However, his symptoms persisted for 10 days. He began to feel pain in his chest when he took a deep breath, and he felt a little out of breath when climbing stairs. David decided to see his doctor.

PERSONAL DETAILS
Name David Palmer
Age 33
Occupation Manager
Family Father died of coronary heart disease. Mother is well.

MEDICAL BACKGROUND
David usually eats a healthy, balanced diet and exercises regularly. He has never smoked and has not had any serious illnesses.

THE CONSULTATION
After David describes his symptoms, his doctor suspects that he might have a viral infection. While listening to his lungs, she can hear a "pleural rub," an abnormal, scratchy sound when David breathes. This sound usually indicates pleurisy, a condition in which the membranes that surround the lungs become inflamed, making it difficult to breathe.

FURTHER INVESTIGATION
The doctor schedules a chest X-ray and blood tests to help identify the cause of David's illness.

The chest X-ray shows some fluffy shadows in the middle of David's right lung, indicating that he has pneumonia. An initial blood test measures the level of antibodies to red blood cells. Exposure to the organism *Mycoplasma pneumoniae* stimulates the immune system to produce these antibodies. More blood tests over the next 3 or 4 weeks will help monitor David's illness.

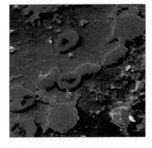

Infecting organism
Mycoplasma pneumoniae *(shown in the color-enhanced photograph above, magnified 20,000 times), a common cause of respiratory tract infections, is the smallest cellular organism known.*

THE DIAGNOSIS
The doctor tells David he has MYCO-PLASMAL PNEUMONIA. Most people with the infection feel well enough to push themselves to continue their normal activities. For this reason, it is often called "walking pneumonia."

THE TREATMENT
While waiting for the results of the blood tests, David's doctor asks him to start taking the antibiotic erythromycin, which is effective against a wide range of bacteria. The doctor also prescribes an anti-inflammatory medication for his chest pain and advises David to take some time off work and to rest. The results of the blood tests confirm the diagnosis and the prescribed course of treatment proves to be effective.

THE OUTCOME
David is able to return to work in a week, but he still has some lingering chest pain and a cough, and feels listless and tired by the end of the day. The symptoms gradually subside until David is back to normal.

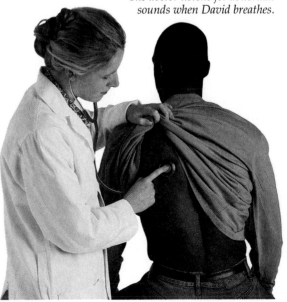

Breathing problems
The doctor listens for abnormal sounds when David breathes.

HEART INFECTIONS

Microorganisms can infect various structures of the heart, especially the valves, causing damage that interferes with heart function (see page 109).

Infective endocarditis

Infective endocarditis can be caused by bacteria or fungi. In infective endocarditis, the organisms infect and damage the heart valves. Acute endocarditis occurs suddenly and can cause sudden tearing of a valve, leading to heart failure (reduced pumping efficiency) and death. The infection produces growths on the valve, which can break apart and lodge in an artery, blocking it or causing small abscesses or bleeding. Endocarditis can also occur in a form that may go undetected for months. Symptoms can include weight loss, lethargy, fever, aching joints, swollen ankles, and breathlessness. The doctor listens for abnormal heart sounds (murmurs) and may order blood cultures and ultrasound images of the heart.

INFECTED HEART VALVES

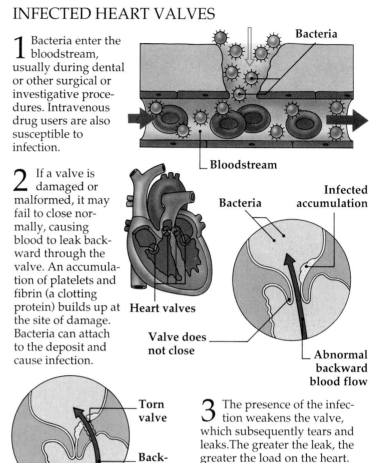

1 Bacteria enter the bloodstream, usually during dental or other surgical or investigative procedures. Intravenous drug users are also susceptible to infection.

Bacteria

Bloodstream

2 If a valve is damaged or malformed, it may fail to close normally, causing blood to leak backward through the valve. An accumulation of platelets and fibrin (a clotting protein) builds up at the site of damage. Bacteria can attach to the deposit and cause infection.

Heart valves

Bacteria

Infected accumulation

Valve does not close

Abnormal backward blood flow

Torn valve

Backward blood flow

3 The presence of the infection weakens the valve, which subsequently tears and leaks. The greater the leak, the greater the load on the heart. The extra stress on the heart can lead to heart failure (a reduction in pumping efficiency).

Preventing bacterial endocarditis
A person with a malformed or artificial heart valve, or a valve that has been damaged by rheumatic heart disease, is susceptible to bacterial endocarditis. The person must inform a dentist or doctor before undergoing invasive procedures. Antibiotics are given before and after all invasive and some investigative procedures.

A person with endocarditis is given intravenous antibiotics or antifungal drugs for several weeks. Severely damaged heart valves may have to be replaced with artificial ones.

Rheumatic heart disease

Rheumatic fever, which mainly affects children and young adults, occurs after infection with streptococcal bacteria. The immune system does not distinguish between the body's own tissues and the bacteria, and produces antibodies that harm its own tissues. Treatment of rheumatic fever involves rest and the anti-inflammatory drug aspirin. The only long-term complication may be damage to heart valves, which makes them susceptible to infections.

SITES OF HEART INFECTIONS

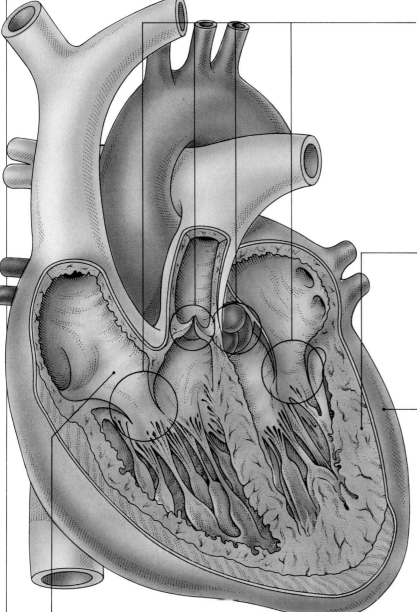

Heart valves
Heart valves normally prevent the backflow of blood inside the heart and are essential for efficient pumping action.

Damaged heart valve
An accumulation of bacteria, platelets, and the protein fibrin (arrow) is shown in the photograph at right. These deposits can break off from the heart valve and block blood vessels in other parts of the body.

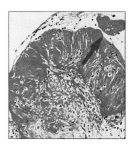

Heart muscle
In myocarditis, the heart muscle becomes inflamed and cannot function efficiently. Myocarditis may be caused by a viral infection or, less commonly, by a parasitic infection. Symptoms include shortness of breath, swollen ankles, irregular heartbeat, and chest pain. Myocarditis usually clears up without treatment but, occasionally, the disorder leads to progressive heart damage.

Pericardium
The pericardium is the two-layered outer covering of the heart.

Pericarditis
Pericarditis, inflammation of the pericardium, may be caused by rheumatic diseases, in which the immune system mistakenly attacks some of the body's own tissues. Pericarditis can also be caused by viruses and, occasionally, by bacteria. Fluid or scar tissue accumulates around the heart and the heart cannot fill with blood (see below). Less blood is pumped out, resulting in a condition that can be fatal. Treatment depends on the cause and on whether the heart has been damaged.

Endocardium
The endocardium is the inside lining of the heart.

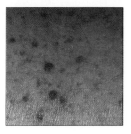

Endocarditis
In bacterial endocarditis, the endocardium and heart valves become inflamed as a result of bacterial infection. Round, purple-red spots called petechiae (left) sometimes occur on mucous membranes or areas of skin.

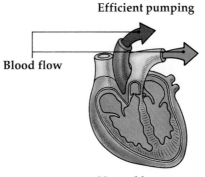

Efficient pumping

Pumping reduced

Blood flow

Normal heart

Pericarditis

Fluid

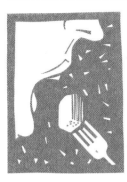

DIGESTIVE TRACT INFECTIONS

I N MANY PARTS OF THE WORLD, digestive tract infections are a major cause of death. Diarrhea, even when not fatal, causes significant illness everywhere. Each year, adults in the US have between one and three bouts of vomiting and diarrhea caused by disease organisms; children have twice as many.

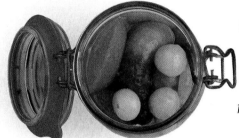

Dangers of contaminated food
Food poisoning is an illness that starts suddenly and can be traced to contaminated food eaten within the previous 2 days. Botulism, usually acquired from improperly preserved food, is a life-threatening form of food poisoning.

Many types of bacteria, viruses, protozoa, and worms can cause illness as a result of their presence or their ability to multiply inside the digestive tract. People usually acquire these infections when they consume food or water that is contaminated with disease organisms.

BACTERIAL INFECTIONS

Infections caused by bacteria are usually easy to treat with antibiotics if the organism is identified quickly. You can avoid some bacterial infections by having vaccinations before visiting high-risk areas.

	INFECTION	SOURCES	SYMPTOMS	TREATMENT
	Typhoid fever	Water or food contaminated by infected feces	High fever; headache; abdominal pain; diarrhea. Incubation: 7 to 14 days. Duration: 4 weeks.	Antibiotics, such as chloramphenicol or ampicillin.
	Salmonellosis	Inadequately cooked animal products; contaminated food	Diarrhea; in severe cases, vomiting; abdominal pain; fever. Incubation: 24 to 48 hours. Duration: About 1 week.	In severe cases requiring hospitalization, antibiotics.
	Shigellosis, also called bacillary dysentery	Person-to-person contact (more common in tropical climates)	Diarrhea with watery stools containing blood and mucus; fever; abdominal pain. Incubation: 24 to 48 hours. Duration: A few days to a week or longer, depending on severity.	Serious infections resulting in hospitalization may require antibiotics and rehydration (see page 114) to replace lost fluids.
	Cholera	Contaminated water or food	Diarrhea. Incubation: 1 to 5 days. Duration: 5 to 7 days; may be fatal.	Rehydration and antibiotics (tetracycline or ampicillin).
	Botulism	Preserved food contaminated with a bacterial toxin	Vomiting; dry mouth; sore throat; breathing problems; numbness; muscle paralysis. Incubation: A few hours to 7 or 8 days. Duration: Fatal in up to 25 percent of cases.	Antitoxin. If a person's breathing fails, he or she is put on a ventilator.
	Campylobacter and *Yersinia* infections	Water or food contaminated by infected feces	Fever; diarrhea; abdominal pain. Incubation: 24 to 72 hours. Duration: 1 week or more.	Antibiotics are given for severe infections.

SITES OF INFECTION

In most cases, digestive tract infections are limited to the intestines, causing diarrhea and vomiting. The resulting loss of fluid can cause dehydration, shock, and even death. Some infections, such as amebiasis, typhoid fever, and salmonellosis, can spread to other parts of the body through the bloodstream.

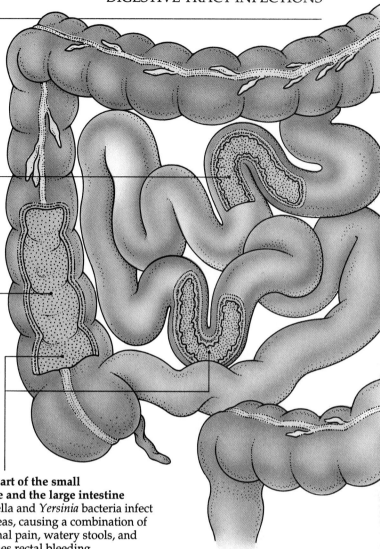

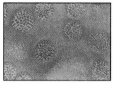

Rotavirus (color-enhanced photograph, magnified 100,000 times)

Small intestine
Rotavirus, Norwalk virus, *Vibrio cholerae* bacteria, and the protozoal parasite *Giardia lamblia* usually infect the small intestine, causing mild abdominal pain and watery stools.

Large intestine
Shigella and *Campylobacter* bacteria and the protozoan *Entamoeba histolytica* infect the large intestine, causing abdominal or rectal pain, smaller than usual stools that contain mucus, and rectal bleeding.

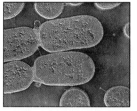

Shigella (color-enhanced photograph, magnified 22,000 times)

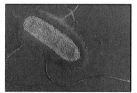

Salmonella enteritidis (color-enhanced photograph, magnified 8,700 times)

Lower part of the small intestine and the large intestine
Salmonella and *Yersinia* bacteria infect these areas, causing a combination of abdominal pain, watery stools, and sometimes rectal bleeding.

VIRAL INFECTIONS

Viruses can enter the intestines and cause infections ranging from a mild stomach upset to severe diarrhea and vomiting. It was not until the 1970s that researchers identified the viruses that attack the intestines specifically. Even today, the causes of 30 to 50 percent of all cases of diarrhea are unknown.

	VIRUS	SOURCES	SYMPTOMS	TREATMENT
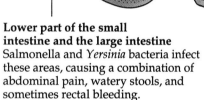	Rotavirus	Contaminated food or water; contact with an infected person	Diarrhea and vomiting; dehydration. Infants and preschool children are most at risk. Incubation period: 1 to 2 days. Duration: 3 to 10 days.	Rehydration (see page 114) and treatment to relieve vomiting and diarrhea.
	Norwalk virus	Contaminated food (usually shellfish) and water	Diarrhea and vomiting. Incubation period: 2 days. Duration: 2 days.	
	Adenovirus	Unknown	Diarrhea; infants are most at risk. Incubation period: Unknown. Duration: Up to 10 days.	

PROTOZOAL INFECTIONS

Protozoa are single-celled animals – microscopic but larger than bacteria – that are often parasites of people. Worldwide, the two most prevalent protozoal infections of the digestive tract are amebiasis and giardiasis (see CASE HISTORY on page 115).

Amebiasis is an infection of the intestines caused by the protozoal parasite *Entamoeba histolytica*. Amebiasis affects an estimated 10 percent of the world's population and nearly one third of people living in some tropical areas. The symptoms of the resulting inflammation of the colon (colitis) include diarrhea and bleeding, abdominal cramps, and weakness. In some people, a liver abscess (see right) develops. Colitis can lead to intestinal bleeding and perforation. Amebiasis is treated with drugs that kill the parasite.

Amebiasis spreads quickly
If amebiasis is not treated quickly, amebae may penetrate the intestines and invade small blood vessels (capillaries). The amebae can then be carried via the portal vein to the liver, where they sometimes produce abscesses. Chills, fever, abdominal pain under the right rib cage, and sudden weight loss are symptoms of a liver abscess.

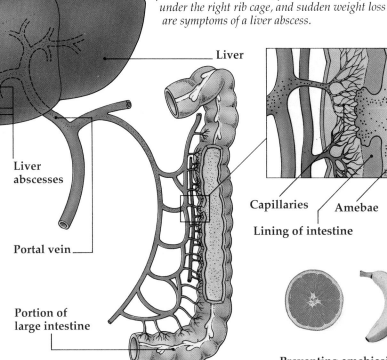

Liver

Liver abscesses

Portal vein

Portion of large intestine

Capillaries   Amebae

Lining of intestine

Preventing amebiasis
Contaminated water and food are the primary sources of amebiasis. If you are visiting a tropical area where the amebae are known to exist, do not eat fresh vegetables or fruit that you cannot peel yourself and do not drink unboiled water.

Cryptosporidiosis

Before 1983, infections caused by the protozoan *Cryptosporidium* were rare. With the AIDS epidemic, the incidence of these infections has increased. People with healthy immune systems occasionally get a mild form of the illness.

Symptoms may include loss of appetite and weight, vomiting, diarrhea, and abdominal pain. However, in people with AIDS, the infection is severe, producing chronic diarrhea and serious weight loss. There are no effective drugs for treating cryptosporidiosis in people with AIDS.

PINWORMS

Pinworm infestations are very common in young children, who can become infested from touching eggs in contaminated food or on clothing or toys and then putting their hands in their mouth. Pinworms lay eggs around the anus, causing irritation. Children often reinfest themselves by scratching the irritation, and then sucking their fingers and swallowing the eggs. A single dose of a worm-fighting drug usually eliminates the worms. The entire household must be treated.

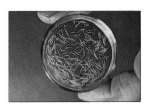

Nighttime irritation
Pinworms (above) usually irritate children at night when the worms come out of the anus to lay eggs. If you examine your child's anal area at night, you can see the threadlike worms.

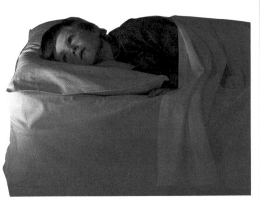

TRAVELERS' DIARRHEA

Each year, an esti-mated 8 million Americans travel to developing coun-tries. Nearly one third of these people will have diarrhea at some time during their trip. Many infections are caused by a local variety of one of the same bacteria that normally inhabit your large intestine.Travelers' diarrhea usu-ally occurs within a couple of days after arriving in a foreign country and lasts for less than 48 hours. You can take several precautions to help reduce your risks (see right).

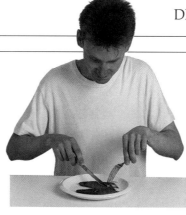

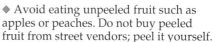

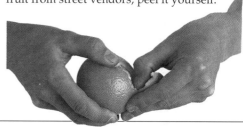

◆ Do not drink unboiled tap water or noncarbonated bottled water or beverages and do not use ice cubes. The acid in carbonated beverages kills disease-causing microbes.

◆ Avoid eating dairy products (including ice cream), shellfish, raw or undercooked meat or fish, un-cooked vegetables, or salads.

◆ Avoid eating unpeeled fruit such as apples or peaches. Do not buy peeled fruit from street vendors; peel it yourself.

WAYS TO PREVENT FOOD POISONING

Food poisoning usually develops after a person eats food contaminated with bacte-ria or their toxins. Occasionally, food poi-soning is caused by viruses, parasites, or toxic chemicals such as those contained in mushrooms.

Health care workers are required to notify local public health departments of out-breaks of food poisoning so that the source of the infection may be found and elimi-nated. You can reduce your risk of food poisoning by following some basic rules.

CAUTION

Food poisoning is usually acquired from food, such as poultry, that has been inadequately defrosted before cooking, not cooked thor-oughly, or im-properly reheated. Raw, contami-nated seafood and insufficiently cooked or raw eggs are also potential sources of food poisoning. Food prepared in unclean kitchens or by people with dirty hands poses a great risk.

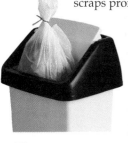

◆ Dispose of table scraps promptly.

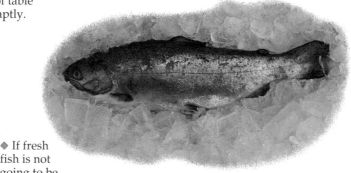

◆ Throw away food that smells bad or is moldy.

◆ Clean utensils and work surfaces be-tween preparations of different food items. Wooden sur-faces should be washed with hot, soapy water and then with a mild solution of chlorine bleach.

◆ Don't leave food uncovered or standing for a long time at room temperature.

◆ If fresh fish is not going to be eaten right away, freeze it.

◆ Refrigerate dairy prod-ucts, such as eggs, milk, and cream.

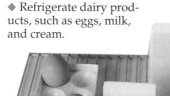

◆ Keep raw meat away from both cooked food and foods that will be served raw.

◆ Eat meat as soon as it has been cooked. Refriger-ate leftovers as quickly as possible after a meal.

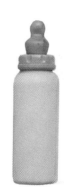

◆ Thoroughly wash baby bottles with dishwashing detergent and hot water before using them.

ASK YOUR DOCTOR
DIGESTIVE TRACT INFECTIONS

Q **I am planning to travel around the world. Are there some areas where I am more likely to get diarrhea?**

A Yes. Certain places, such as Africa, Asia, Latin America, and southern Europe have high rates of endemic (always present in the population) infections caused by parasitic worms, protozoa, bacteria, and viruses. These organisms cause diarrhea in 20 to 50 percent of travelers to those areas. Before you leave on your trip, ask your doctor what you can do to avoid getting sick. Taking bismuth subsalicylate tablets daily while traveling can substantially reduce your risk of diarrhea.

Q **Are antibiotics necessary to treat diarrhea? What is the risk of spreading infection?**

A Antibiotics are necessary only in severe cases. If you follow basic rules of hygiene, such as washing your hands after using the toilet and before preparing food, there is only a small risk that you will spread your infection to others.

Q **What should I do if I get a digestive tract infection while on vacation? Should I cancel the rest of my trip and come home?**

A In most healthy adults, a stomach upset and diarrhea are not serious medical problems. Drink plenty of fluids and eat a bland diet until your symptoms disappear. In severe cases, you should see a doctor. Infants, the elderly, and people with chronic diseases such as diabetes are more at risk. Discuss your concerns with your doctor before you leave.

REHYDRATION FOR DIARRHEA

If diarrhea is severe, fluids and salts lost from the intestines must be replaced with a rehydration solution. You can buy premixed ingredients that you mix with water or you can make your own solution (see below). A dehydrated person should drink 2 to 3 pints of rehydration solution every few hours until his or her condition improves. If dehydration is severe, or if the person cannot take fluids by mouth because of nausea or vomiting, an intravenous infusion in a hospital may be required.

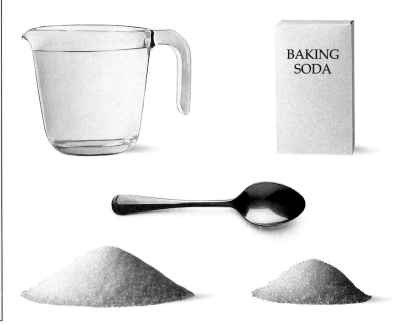

Preparing an oral rehydration solution
Make your own rehydration solution to treat dehydration by adding ¹/₂ teaspoon of salt, 2 tablespoons of sugar, and ¹/₂ teaspoon of baking soda to 1 pint of water. Discard any solution that has not been used within 24 hours and prepare a new mixture.

BAKING SODA

WHEN SHOULD YOU CONSULT A DOCTOR?

If you have mild diarrhea and vomiting, your symptoms will probably subside in 12 to 24 hours. However, if you have severe watery diarrhea, which can cause dehydration, seek medical attention immediately. Your doctor will advise you about fluid intake and how to treat the diarrhea and other symptoms. Symptoms of dehydration include thirst, dizziness, and fainting.

CASE HISTORY
DIARRHEA AND BLOATING

JOE HAD A TERRIFIC time at summer camp. A week or so after he returned, he began to feel sick and had diarrhea and an uncomfortable sensation of bloating in his abdomen. He also had occasional cramps. Joe's mother was worried about his loss of appetite, especially when he started to lose weight. She made an appointment for Joe to see his doctor.

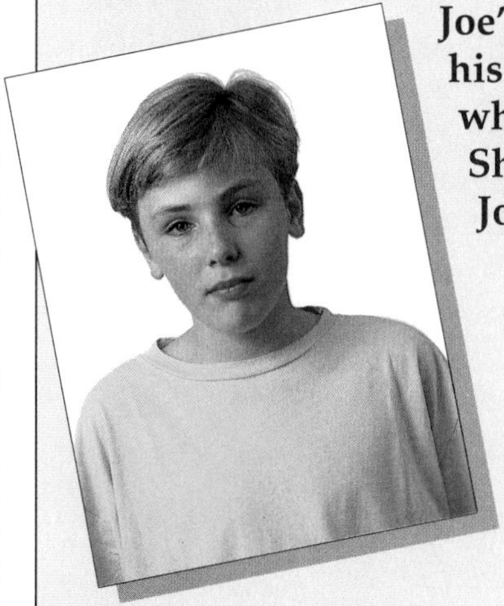

PERSONAL DETAILS
Name Joe Haldane
Age 14
Occupation High school student
Family Father has high blood pressure. Mother and younger sister are both well.

MEDICAL BACKGROUND
Joe had chickenpox when he was 6 years old and fractured his left arm when he was 9. Otherwise, he has been very healthy.

THE CONSULTATION
The doctor asks Joe about his symptoms, his activities at camp, what he ate and drank while at camp, and whether any of the other boys who went to the camp are now sick. Joe tells his doctor that one day during a hike he drank water from a mountain stream. The doctor performs a physical examination and determines that the most likely explanation for Joe's symptoms is an intestinal infection. She asks Joe to provide a sample of feces to send to the laboratory for analysis. The results of the analysis will help her make a diagnosis of Joe's illness.

THE DIAGNOSIS
The laboratory analysis of Joe's feces shows that it contains microscopic *Giardia lamblia* protozoal parasites, indicating that he has GIARDIASIS. The doctor explains to Joe and his mother that giardiasis is an intestinal infection that can occur when a person drinks water that is contaminated with the parasites. She tells Joe that he probably contracted the infection when he drank water from the mountain stream. She says that wild animals such as beavers, which can carry the infection, may have contaminated the stream.

THE TREATMENT
The doctor explains that this type of intestinal infection usually does not get better without treatment. She prescribes an antibiotic (metronidazole) to be taken for a short period of time that will act against parasites. The doctor tells Joe that his symptoms should clear up completely. However, if the infection is not eliminated, Joe will need to take another course of the medication.

THE OUTLOOK
Joe starts to feel better right away, although he still feels a little bloated and he does not gain weight for a couple of weeks. By the time school starts in the fall, Joe's digestive system is back to normal.

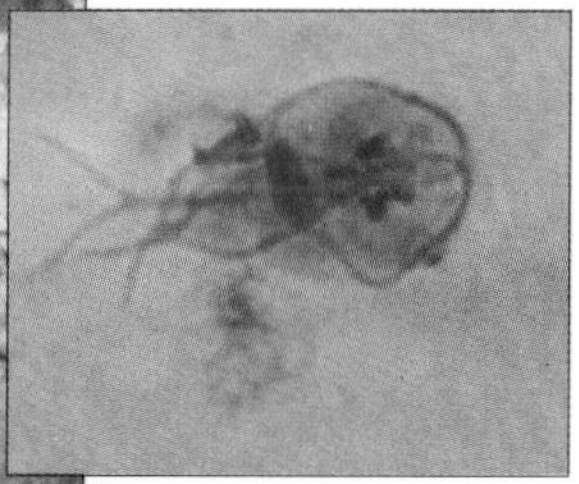

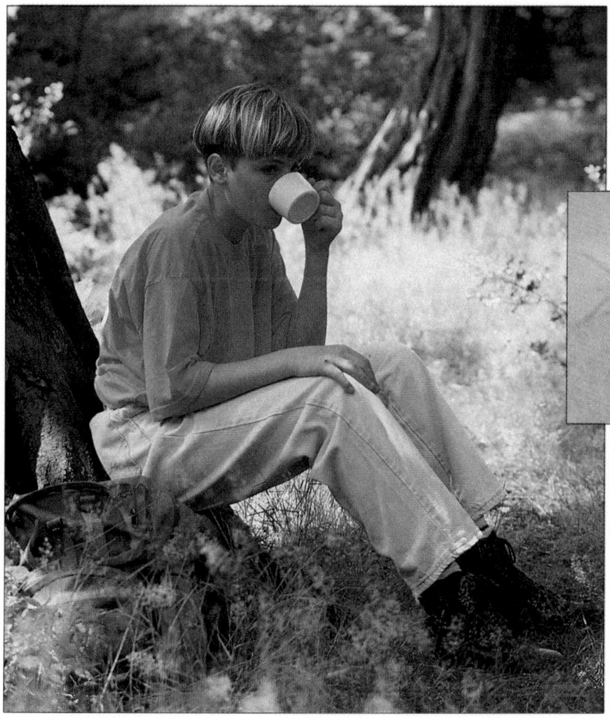

Contaminated drinking water
Wild animals can contaminate streams by spreading protozoal parasites such as Giardia lamblia *(shown above, magnified 1,300 times).*

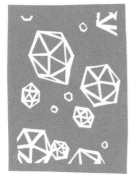

VIRAL HEPATITIS

HEPATITIS IS A common and serious illness that is caused by several different viruses – including the hepatitis A, B, C, and D viruses. The incidence of acute viral hepatitis has been slowly rising in the US during the last 20 years. The hepatitis viruses infect the liver, causing inflammation.

One function of the liver is to remove toxic substances from the bloodstream and process them so they can be excreted from the body. If the liver becomes infected, as it does in cases of viral hepatitis, it cannot work properly. As a result, toxic substances build up in the bloodstream, with the potential to cause serious illness. Other important functions of the liver (see WHAT YOUR LIVER DOES on page 117) may also be impaired.

TYPES OF INFECTIONS

Hepatitis infections are classified as acute or chronic. The symptoms of acute hepatitis occur suddenly and may be severe, and the outcome of the infection can usually be determined within 6 weeks. A person either recovers completely, recovers with some liver damage, or, in rare cases, dies. However, if the inflammation continues indefinitely, the illness can take one of two forms – chronic active or chronic persistent hepatitis. Chronic active hepatitis leads to death; chronic persistent hepatitis, which causes little damage to the liver (see page 118), is not life-threatening.

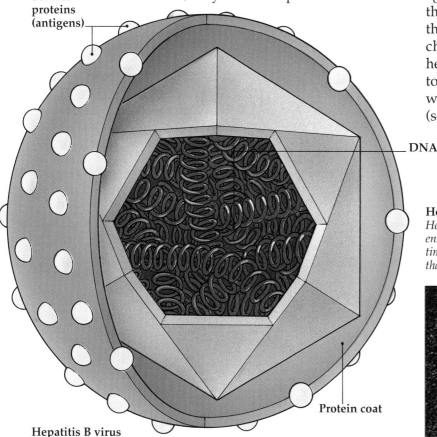

Surface proteins (antigens)

DNA

Protein coat

Hepatitis B virus
The Dane particle (shown above) – one form of the hepatitis B virus – is a small, 20-sided structure with a protein coat that encloses the virus's genetic material (DNA). Surface proteins (called antigens) that are attached to this coat sometimes help doctors identify the virus in a person's blood.

Hepatitis A virus
Hepatitis A virus particles (shown in the color-enhanced photograph below, magnified 230,000 times) are small, 20-sided encapsulated structures that contain DNA (genetic material).

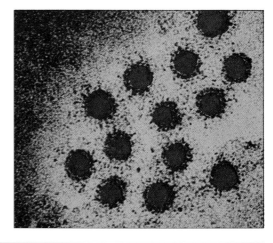

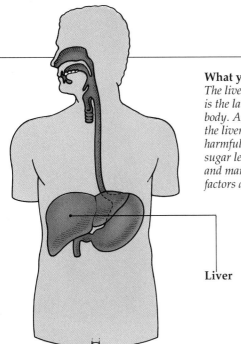

What your liver does
The liver, located in your abdomen, is the largest organ inside your body. Among its many functions, the liver stores nutrients, detoxifies harmful substances, maintains blood sugar levels, facilitates digestion, and manufactures blood clotting factors and other important proteins.

Liver

The hepatitis D, or delta, virus causes disease only when it occurs simultaneously with a hepatitis B infection or in people who have chronic hepatitis B. However, when it does occur, delta hepatitis is usually a very severe illness.

ACUTE HEPATITIS

Bed rest is the only treatment for acute hepatitis types B and C. A person's immune system produces antibodies to fight the virus. In severe cases, the infections may cause liver failure, which can be fatal. A liver transplant may be considered for a person with liver failure.

HEPATITIS VIRUSES

An estimated 40 percent of young adults in urban areas of the US and almost all children in developing countries have been exposed to the hepatitis A virus. The virus usually causes only a mild illness from which nearly all infected people recover completely. Hepatitis A is common in preschool children, most of whom do not have any symptoms.

Each year, approximately 300,000 people in the US acquire hepatitis B. The time between exposure to the virus and development of symptoms can be as long as 4 months. About 10 percent of people with hepatitis B become seriously ill, but in healthy adults the death rate is less than 1 percent. One out of 10 people with hepatitis B develops chronic hepatitis, which can lead to cirrhosis of the liver or liver cancer.

Until hepatitis C was identified in 1989, it was included in a group of hepatitis viruses defined by what they were not – non-A, non-B hepatitis. Before the blood test for hepatitis C recently became available, the virus was the most frequent cause of transfusion-related hepatitis. The symptoms of acute hepatitis C usually are less severe than those of hepatitis B, but hepatitis C is more likely to become chronic and lead to cirrhosis.

SYMPTOMS AND SIGNS OF HEPATITIS

The early symptoms of viral hepatitis can be vague. A person with hepatitis may have loss of appetite, nausea and vomiting, aching joints and muscles, headache, sensitivity to light, coughing, a sore throat, a runny nose, and a mild fever. Within 1 to 2 weeks, however, jaundice may develop (see below) and the nausea and loss of appetite may become more severe. The person may still have a slight fever.

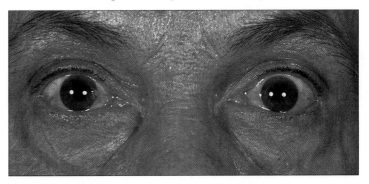

What is jaundice?
Jaundice is the accumulation in the bloodstream of bilirubin, a pigment produced by the breakdown of red blood cells. Normally, the liver removes bilirubin from the blood, modifies it, and excretes it in the feces. But in a person with hepatitis, the liver stops working properly, causing bilirubin to build up in the blood. The accumulation of bilirubin produces a yellow tint in the whites of the eyes (above) and the skin.

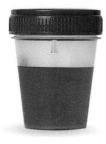

Dark urine
In a person with hepatitis, bilirubin that has not been processed completely by the liver builds up in the bloodstream and enters the urine, turning it dark (left). The feces become pale or even white because bilirubin does not reach the intestines.

HOW VIRAL HEPATITIS IS TRANSMITTED

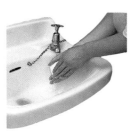

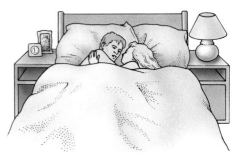

Contaminated food and water
A person with hepatitis A excretes the virus in urine and feces. Hepatitis A is transmitted through contaminated food, water, and contact with contaminated objects, particularly in areas where sanitation is poor.

Sexual intercourse
Virus particles are present in the body fluids – blood, saliva, and semen – of a person with hepatitis B, C, or D and can be transmitted during sexual intercourse.

Blood transfusions
Because there are blood tests to identify the hepatitis B and C viruses, these viruses are now rarely transmitted through blood transfusions.

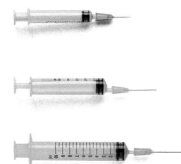

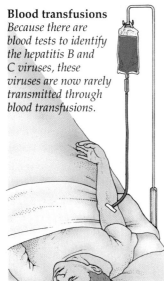

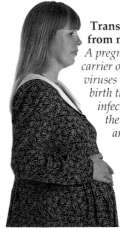

Transmission from mother to baby
A pregnant woman who is a carrier of the hepatitis B, C, or D viruses can infect her baby at birth through contact with infected body fluids. Giving the infant an injection of antibodies and a vaccination at birth prevents the baby from developing hepatitis B.

Needle-stick injuries and contaminated needles and syringes
Hepatitis types B, C, and D can all be transmitted through blood-to-blood contact. Infection can occur in health-care workers as a result of a needle-stick injury, or in drug addicts who use unsterilized, contaminated needles and syringes.

CHRONIC HEPATITIS

A substantial percentage of people infected with the hepatitis B or C virus develop chronic hepatitis – either an active or persistent form of the infection. In chronic active hepatitis, the person either does not recover from the initial attack, or symptoms develop without any obvious acute illness. Symptoms include fatigue, loss of appetite, a slight fever, and, usually, jaundice. Without treatment, the disease can progress for several years until cirrhosis of the liver or, in some cases, liver cancer develops. Complications resulting from cirrhosis and liver cancer can be fatal. However, treatment with corticosteroids (anti-inflammatory drugs) and interferon (an antiviral agent) has improved the outlook for people with this condition.

In chronic persistent hepatitis, inflammation of the liver continues after the initial infection. The inflammation may clear up after a few years, and damage to the liver, if any, is usually slight. However, the person may still be a carrier of the virus and may be able to infect others.

PROTECTION AGAINST INFECTION

There is no vaccine for hepatitis A, but Americans planning to visit developing countries can ask their doctor if they should have an injection of immune globulin, which is rich in human antibodies to the hepatitis A virus. The protection provided by the antibodies usually lasts about 2 to 6 months.

Effective vaccines are available for the hepatitis B virus (see box at right). Currently, there is no vaccine for hepatitis C.

VACCINATION AGAINST HEPATITIS B

Vaccination is recommended for anyone who is at increased risk of infection, such as health-care workers, children of women who are carriers, and people (including hemophiliacs) who require repeated blood transfusions. Immunity to hepatitis B provides protection against both the B and D viruses.

CASE HISTORY
LOSS OF ENERGY AND APPETITE

OSCAR USUALLY WOKE UP **easily on Saturday mornings to go jogging. However, one Saturday, he just didn't have the energy. Over the next 2 weeks he had less and less energy and lost interest in food. After Oscar's wife noticed that his skin looked yellow, he went to see his doctor at the hospital where he works.**

PERSONAL DETAILS
Name Oscar Hernandez
Age 37
Occupation Laboratory technician
Family Both of Oscar's parents are living. His mother takes medication for high blood pressure.

MEDICAL BACKGROUND
Oscar enjoys sports, stays in shape, and usually has a healthy appetite. Other than childhood illnesses and some minor sports injuries, he has not had any medical problems.

THE CONSULTATION
Oscar tells the doctor that he feels nauseated after meals. The doctor finds that Oscar has a raised temperature and an enlarged and tender liver. Oscar's skin and the whites of his eyes have a yellow tint (jaundice) and a specimen of his urine is dark. Oscar also tells his doctor that his bowel movements look pale. These are all signs of liver inflammation.

The doctor asks Oscar if he can recall any time recently that a used needle or any other sharp medical instrument penetrated his skin. Oscar remembers that, about 4 months ago, he helped clean up some broken glass in the laboratory after a rack of blood sample vials fell on the floor. The doctor asks Oscar if he has received the vaccination now recom-mended for hospital workers as protection against the hepatitis B virus. Oscar recalls that someone suggested he have the hepatitis B vaccination last year, but he never did.

THE DIAGNOSIS
Because of Oscar's jaundice, weakness, and nausea, he is admitted to the hospital for a series of blood tests and tests to check the function of his

Blood tests
In the hospital, Oscar has a series of blood tests to check the function of his liver and to look for antibodies to hepatitis B. He also has a blood test to determine whether his immune system has produced antibodies to HIV, the virus that causes AIDS. The HIV blood test will be repeated in 2 months and again in 8 months.

liver. The results show that Oscar has VIRAL HEPATITIS B. Because of the possibility that he may have been infected with the human immuno-deficiency virus (HIV) – the virus that causes AIDS – from the spilled blood, the doctor recommends that Oscar have a blood test for antibodies to HIV. The doctor suggests that his wife also have the tests, because both hepatitis B and HIV can be transmitted sexually. The doctor recommends that, until Oscar's last HIV test (in about 8 months), the couple use condoms during sex.

THE TREATMENT
There is no treatment for viral hepa-titis other than rest. Oscar begins to feel better after 10 days. As soon as his liver starts to heal, he is sent home. His wife's tests indicate that she has not been infected with the hepatitis virus. As a precaution, she is given an injection of antibodies, to be repeated in 30 days. Neither Os-car nor his wife appears to have been infected with HIV.

THE OUTCOME
After 2 more weeks, Oscar is able to return to work. He must continue to have blood tests until the results show that the hepatitis infection has completely subsided. The doctor also recommends that Oscar be tested for HIV in 2 months and again in 8 months.

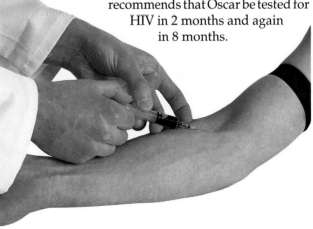

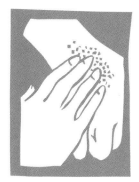

SKIN INFECTIONS AND INFESTATIONS

AN ASSORTMENT OF MICROORGANISMS can infect the skin. Parasites can live on the surface of the body and cause irritation by biting or burrowing into the skin. Some infections and infestations of parasites cause few or no symptoms but others can change your appearance and cause pain, itching, and swelling. Few skin infections or infestations, however, create serious problems if they are treated at an early stage.

Infections of the skin are common, even in healthy people. Many factors can increase your susceptibility. If you are taking certain kinds of drugs, have a serious illness such as diabetes, or have an existing skin condition or open sore, you are more at risk for skin problems. Being overweight with overlapping rolls of skin, or even living in a hot, moist climate, can also increase your risk of having a skin disorder.

BACTERIAL INFECTIONS

In general, bacterial infections of the skin can be avoided by good personal hygiene. Still, some bacterial skin infections such as acne are relatively common.

Acne

Many adolescents and some adults have acne, a condition characterized by inflammation and infection of the hair follicles and the sebaceous glands in the skin, which secrete a lubricant called sebum. The most common type of acne – acne vulgaris – is associated with an excessive production of sebum. A high level of sebum production may result from elevated levels of sex hormones. Because acne often runs in families, it is thought that increased sebum secretion may be genetically linked.

There is no simple cure for acne but most cases improve by the time a person

CONTROLLING ACNE

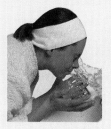

◆ Wash your face twice daily with an antibacterial soap but don't irritate your skin by scrubbing too hard.

◆ Apply an anti-acne preparation that contains benzoyl peroxide to affected areas of your skin to open pores and release trapped sebum (oil).

◆ Wash your hair regularly and keep it off your face. Oil in hair often aggravates acne.

◆ Avoid oil-based cosmetics and skin-care products.

◆ Don't pick or squeeze blemishes. This can spread infection to deeper layers of the skin and increase the risk of scarring.

◆ Consult your doctor if your acne persists.

HOW ACNE DEVELOPS

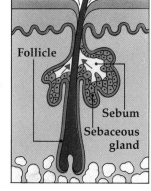

Normal follicles
The sebaceous glands secrete sebum, an oil that lubricates the hair and skin. In normal skin, sebum flows unobstructed from the hair follicles (pores).

Hair

Follicle

Sebum

Sebaceous gland

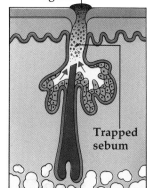

Plug

Trapped sebum

Blackheads
Hair follicles can become blocked by dead skin cells and sebum, forming a hardened plug. Exposure to oxygen in the air turns the plug black.

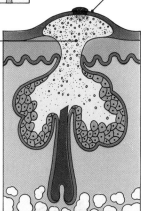

Inflammation

Pus

Infected follicles
Sebum and skin cells trapped inside a blocked hair follicle may become infected by bacteria normally found in the skin, resulting in the inflammation and pus that often accompany acne pustules, cysts, and nodules.

Acne vulgaris
Acne vulgaris, shown here, occurs most frequently during adolescence on areas of the skin that have a high concentration of sebaceous (oil) glands. The face is affected most often – particularly the forehead, nose, and chin – but pimples may also form on the neck, shoulders, back, or chest.

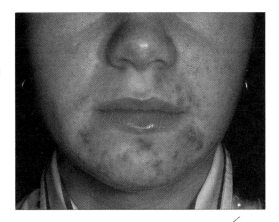

reaches his or her mid-20s. Mild acne can often be controlled with skin medications containing benzoyl peroxide and other measures (see CONTROLLING ACNE on page 120). Moderate to severe cases are often treated with antibiotics. Severe acne can be treated with retinoid drugs, which help to prevent scarring. These synthetic compounds are chemically related to vitamin A, which plays an important role in maintaining healthy cells.

Boils and carbuncles

Infected hair follicles or sebaceous glands can also result in the formation of a painful, pus-filled swelling (boil) or a cluster of interconnected boils (carbuncle). Both boils and carbuncles are more common in people who do not bathe regularly and in people with weakened immune systems or diabetes.

Bursting a boil can spread the infection. Applying hot compresses every 2 hours helps drain the pus and relieves pain and swelling. Sometimes carbuncles or very large boils have to be cut open and drained. Antibiotics are given in severe cases.

How a boil develops
A boil, shown at left and below, may develop when certain types of bacteria enter a hair follicle. In reaction to the infection, the skin becomes inflamed and the hair follicle fills with pus. The resulting swelling can be extremely painful. Boils are more common in moist areas of the body, such as the groin, the back of the neck, the armpits, and the area around the anus. In most people, boils are caused by the bacterium Staphylococcus aureus.

CROSS SECTION OF A BOIL

Normal hair follicle

Hair

Sebaceous gland

Inflammation

Sebaceous gland

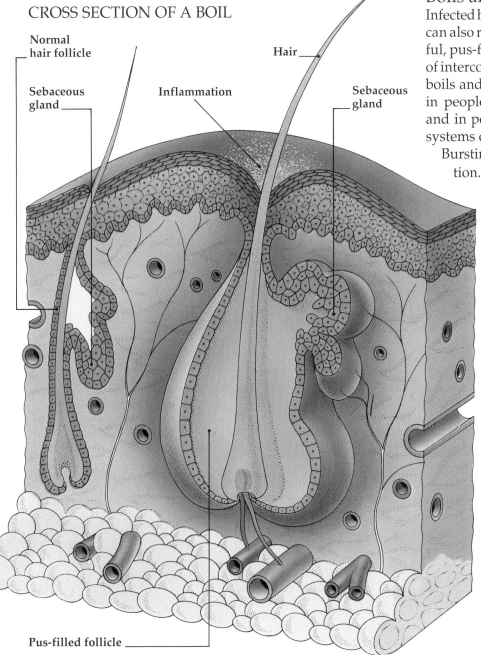

Pus-filled follicle

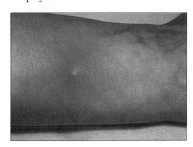

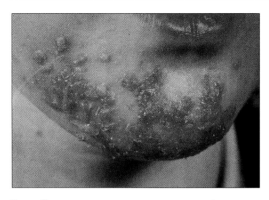

Impetigo
This highly contagious condition is characterized by small, fluid-filled blisters that usually appear around the nose and mouth. The blisters tend to burst so quickly that they are seldom noticed. A bursting blister releases fluid that forms honey-colored crusts over the area (see above). The crusts can be removed by soaking them with warm salt water.

Infection in broken skin

When bacteria enter a break in the skin, the area may become inflamed. Occasionally, more serious skin disorders such as impetigo, erysipelas, or cellulitis develop. These skin infections are usually caused by streptococcal or staphylococcal bacteria. Erysipelas affects only the upper layers of the skin, but cellulitis and streptococcal impetigo can affect deeper tissues. These infections can be treated with antibiotics.

VIRAL INFECTIONS

The most common viral infections of the skin are caused by different types of herpesviruses or papillomaviruses.

Herpes simplex infections

Infections caused by the herpes simplex virus are characterized by small, fluid-filled blisters and can vary from mild disorders to life-threatening illnesses. Like other infections, herpes infections are most serious in people whose immune systems are weakened.

The herpes simplex virus (see page 49) can be spread by direct contact with an open herpes sore. Genital herpes can also be spread by contact with body fluids such as vaginal secretions. The herpes simplex virus can cause recurrent sores on an infected person's lips (cold sores) or in the genital area (see GENITAL HERPES on page 131).

Once infection occurs, the virus remains in the body for life. The initial infection, which most often affects people in childhood or early adult life, causes the most severe symptoms. Recurrent infections are usually milder.

(see page 49) ... (see GENITAL HERPES on page 131).

TREATING HERPES

First-time genital herpes infections can be treated with the antiviral drug acyclovir in an ointment form. The drug helps relieve symptoms and speeds healing of the blisters. Long-term use of acyclovir capsules may decrease the frequency and severity of outbreaks in people who have numerous and severe recurrences. Cold sores are treated with an over-the-counter ointment. Recurrences may be triggered by sunlight, other illnesses, stress, or the menstrual cycle. Using number 15 sunscreen helps prevent recurrent cold sores.

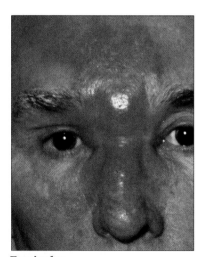

Erysipelas
Erysipelas often begins suddenly with a fever, headache, and vomiting. The affected skin becomes itchy and develops into a red, swollen area with a sharply defined border, as shown above. Lymph glands may also become swollen.

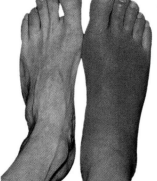

Herpetic whitlow
In addition to causing sores around the lips or on the genitals, the herpes simplex virus may cause blisters to form on the fingers, as shown above. This infection is known as herpetic whitlow. It usually occurs in people such as doctors or dentists who are exposed to sores or secretions from the nose, lips, or mouth.

Cellulitis
Cellulitis (shown here on the right foot) most frequently involves the face, neck, or legs. The affected area is red, raised, hot, and tender, and is larger and less well-defined than in erysipelas. A high fever, chills, and tender, swollen lymph glands are common symptoms of cellulitis.

Excess cells

Epidermis
(outer layer
of skin)

Dermis
(inner layer
of skin)

External lump

How a wart grows
The human papilloma-
virus enters the skin
through small cuts
and causes cells in the
epidermis (the outer
layer of skin) to
multiply. Increased
numbers of cells may
push upward to form a
firm, raised lump on
the skin's surface or
may be pushed inward
in areas subject to
constant pressure such
as the soles of the feet.

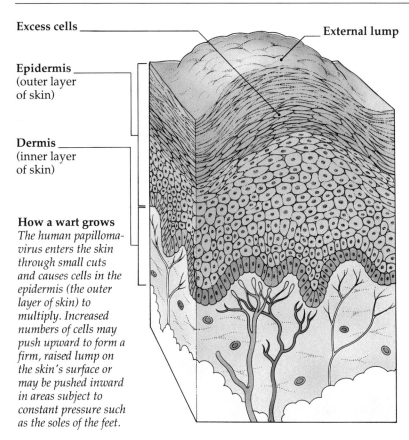

Common warts
The warts on this
person's thumb are
common warts, which
grow in areas of the
body subject to injury,
such as the face, hands,
or knees. Injury reduces
the ability of tissues to
ward off infection.
Children are most
frequently affected.

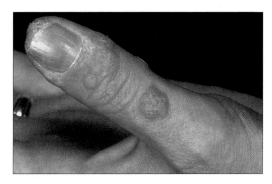

Warts

Warts are benign (noncancerous) tumors of the skin or mucous membranes caused by a wide range of human papillomaviruses. The areas of the body that are affected and the appearance of the warts depend on the type of human papillomavirus involved. (Genital warts are discussed on page 132.) Because they can be spread by direct contact, warts often appear in clusters on the skin. There is nothing you can do to avoid them. Treatment of warts depends on where

they are on the body. Many warts disappear within 3 to 6 months, but some can be removed more quickly by your doctor with salicylic acid. Particularly stubborn warts can be removed using a freezing technique or they can be burned or scraped off after administration of a local anesthetic.

FUNGAL INFECTIONS

Fungal infections are usually confined to the mucous membranes, the outer layers of the skin, or the nails. Most are caused by either dermatophyte or *Candida* organisms (see FUNGI on page 52).

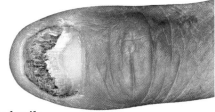

Infected nails
This photograph shows a fingernail infected by
dermatophyte fungi. Infected nails are particularly
difficult to treat and often must be removed.

Common infections

A group of dermatophyte fungi causes some common infections of the skin, hair, and nails that can be spread by direct contact with an infected person or animal or with contaminated objects such as towels, socks, or combs. The most common of these infections is athletes' foot, which causes cracking and itching of the skin between the toes. Ringworm is characterized by red, circular patches on the skin. Jock itch, which primarily affects males, produces a red, itchy rash in the groin around the genitals.

Dermatophyte infections are diagnosed by examining scrapings of skin under a microscope, sometimes using ultraviolet light, which makes some fungi become fluorescent. Mild infections can be cleared up with antifungal preparations applied to the skin, but more serious infections may require antifungal medication taken by mouth.

VAGINAL YEAST
INFECTIONS

Vaginal yeast infections, which often recur, can be triggered by pregnancy, serious illness, stress, antibiotics, or the oral contraceptive pill. To prevent repeated attacks:

◆ Use antifungal medications, which are now available over-the-counter.

◆ Wear cotton underwear and loose clothing to help keep the vaginal area dry.

◆ Consider switching from oral contraceptives to another form of birth control.

◆ Don't take antibiotics unnecessarily. Antibiotics can kill bacteria normally present in the body, permitting yeast organisms to grow.

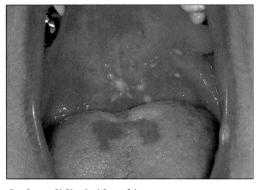

Oral candidiasis (thrush)
Candida *infections in the mouth, which are common, produce sore, raised, cream-colored or red patches on the surface of the tongue or on the mucous membranes of the mouth (shown above).*

Yeast infection

The yeast *Candida albicans,* and other *Candida* organisms, can infect the mucous membranes and moist areas of the skin. The yeast infection called candidiasis usually occurs on the mucous membranes inside the vagina or mouth or on the tip of the penis (see page 52). Yeast infections can be acquired through sexual contact but usually originate in the infected person's body. Women are affected by candidiasis more often than men. Most yeast infections respond rapidly to antifungal medications.

SKIN INFESTATIONS

Most parasite infestations in people involve the burrowing mite *Sarcoptes scabiei* or lice (see LICE AND MITES on page 59). Infestation by *Sarcoptes scabiei,* known as scabies, is highly contagious and is transmitted by close person-to-person contact or, sometimes, by an animal. It affects all socioeconomic groups but is more prevalent among people living in crowded, unclean conditions or in institutions such as prisons. The primary symptom of scabies is an intense itching that develops about 3 or 4 weeks after initial infestation. The itching is usually worse at night and after bathing.

Three kinds of lice are parasites of people, feeding on their blood. Head lice infest the head and pubic lice mainly infest the genital area. Pubic lice are transmitted primarily during sexual contact (see CRAB LICE on page 134). Body lice feed on blood but live in clothing. Head and pubic lice can affect anyone but body lice are most often found in people living in unclean conditions who seldom wash or change their clothes.

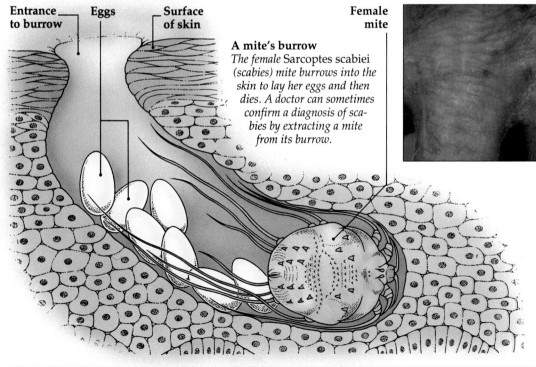

| Entrance to burrow | Eggs | Surface of skin | Female mite |

A mite's burrow
The female Sarcoptes scabiei *(scabies) mite burrows into the skin to lay her eggs and then dies. A doctor can sometimes confirm a diagnosis of scabies by extracting a mite from its burrow.*

Signs of scabies
The burrowing of female scabies mites often produces scaly swellings of the skin like those visible on the skin between the fingers pictured above. Scratching the skin can spread the infection.

DESTROYING LICE AND SCABIES MITES

Lice infestations and scabies are treated with insecticides that kill the parasites and their eggs. You should use these products with caution because they can irritate the mucous membranes or inflame the skin when used excessively. Some insecticides should not be used to treat infestations in pregnant women or infants. Wash and dry bedding and clothing at high temperatures to make sure that parasites are removed. Boil all hairbrushes, combs, and hair ornaments. If hats cannot be washed, throw them away. You can avoid the spread of head lice by not sharing combs, hairbrushes, or hats.

Using insecticidal shampoo or creme rinse
Apply the shampoo or creme rinse to hair and massage it into the scalp. Make sure the lather does not drip into the eyes or mouth. Leave the shampoo or creme rinse on for the recommended length of time – usually 5 to 10 minutes – and then rinse the hair thoroughly. Use a fine-toothed comb to remove dead lice and eggs. Boil all hairbrushes and combs to kill any eggs or lice. Repeat the treatment if necessary.

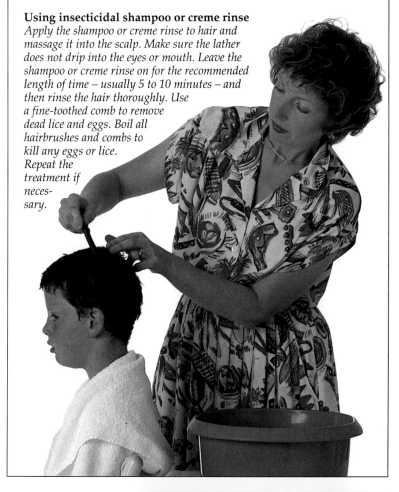

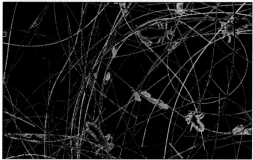

Head lice
Adult lice and their eggs, shown here on human hair at just over twice life size, are visible to the naked eye. Lice can cause intense itching of the scalp and inflammation of the skin, especially at the nape of the neck and behind the ears.

ASK YOUR DOCTOR
SKIN INFECTIONS AND INFESTATIONS

Q **I keep getting boils on the back of my neck. What can I do about them?**

A Recurrent boils sometimes indicate the presence of some disorder that weakens resistance to infections. Your doctor may want to test you for diabetes or an impaired immune system. You may be advised to wash your skin daily with an antibacterial soap and to take showers instead of baths. Bacteria from the boil can accumulate in bath water and spread to other areas of your skin.

Q **My daughter has several small, smooth, flesh-colored bumps on her skin, each with a tiny hole. What caused them?**

A Your daughter may have molluscum contagiosum, a harmless skin infection caused by a pox virus. The infection is transmitted by direct contact with an infected person and is more common among children than adults. Avoid touching the bumps and ask your doctor to examine them. The infection usually clears up within a few months without treatment.

Q **A few weeks ago I used an insecticidal lotion to treat scabies but I have it again. Why didn't the treatment work?**

A Only one or two applications of insecticide are necessary to kill scabies mites but, unless all household members are treated at the same time, the infestation can recur. Anyone you come into close contact with should also be treated. Launder all linens in soap and very hot water and change and wash your clothes often.

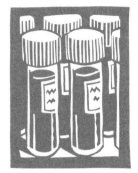

URINARY TRACT INFECTIONS

U SUALLY, the free, unobstructed flow of urine and your body's defenses prevent microorganisms that naturally inhabit your body from infecting your urinary tract. A urinary tract infection occurs when organisms enter the urethra (the tube that carries urine from the bladder to outside the body) and multiply there or move up to the bladder or kidneys.

DIABETES MELLITUS

Infections of the urinary tract are more common in people with diabetes mellitus because this chronic illness impairs the immune system. Poor control of diabetes increases the risk of acquiring infections.

Most of the microorganisms that cause urinary tract infections spread to the urethra from around the anus. Women are at higher risk for these infections than men because the female urethra is very short and the opening is much closer to the anus, which allows organisms easier access to the bladder.

Urinary tract infections in people under 50
Urinary tract infections are extremely common in women but rare in men until after age 50. Although uncommon in infants, urinary tract infections can have serious consequences when they occur in babies. The incidence of urinary tract infections in girls increases significantly with the onset of adolescence and with sexual activity.

CAUSES OF URINARY TRACT INFECTION

Anything that prevents the bladder from emptying completely – such as stones in the bladder, kidney, or ureter (the tube that carries urine from the kidney to the bladder) – makes infection more likely. Other factors that influence your risk of acquiring an infection vary according to your age and sex.

Urinary tract infections in older people
Older people are at high risk of infection because they have lowered resistance and may have medical problems that interfere with the outflow of urine. These problems include an enlarged prostate gland in men and a relaxation of the muscles supporting the bladder in women.

PERCENTAGE OF PEOPLE WITH URINARY TRACT INFECTIONS

- Infants; preschoolers
- Children; adolescents
- Adults
- Pregnant women
- Older people

0.03 – 0.06%

1 – 1.9%

0.05%

2.5%

0.2 – 0.6%

0.4 – 2.7%

2 – 11%

2 – 15%

15 – 20%

SITES OF URINARY TRACT INFECTION

The symptoms and consequences of urinary tract infections depend on the site of infection. Infections in the lower part of the urinary tract (the bladder and urethra) are more common and less serious than those that spread to the kidney. Kidney infections can cause serious and permanent damage.

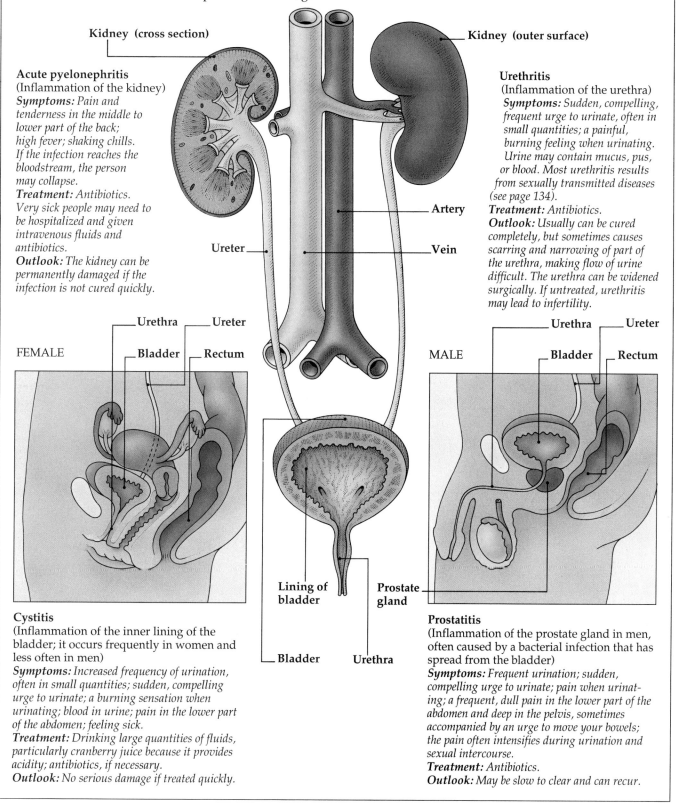

Kidney (cross section)

Kidney (outer surface)

Acute pyelonephritis
(Inflammation of the kidney)
Symptoms: Pain and tenderness in the middle to lower part of the back; high fever; shaking chills. If the infection reaches the bloodstream, the person may collapse.
Treatment: Antibiotics. Very sick people may need to be hospitalized and given intravenous fluids and antibiotics.
Outlook: The kidney can be permanently damaged if the infection is not cured quickly.

Urethritis
(Inflammation of the urethra)
Symptoms: Sudden, compelling, frequent urge to urinate, often in small quantities; a painful, burning feeling when urinating. Urine may contain mucus, pus, or blood. Most urethritis results from sexually transmitted diseases (see page 134).
Treatment: Antibiotics.
Outlook: Usually can be cured completely, but sometimes causes scarring and narrowing of part of the urethra, making flow of urine difficult. The urethra can be widened surgically. If untreated, urethritis may lead to infertility.

Artery

Ureter

Vein

Urethra   **Ureter**

FEMALE

Bladder   **Rectum**

Urethra   **Ureter**

MALE

Bladder   **Rectum**

Lining of bladder

Prostate gland

Bladder   **Urethra**

Cystitis
(Inflammation of the inner lining of the bladder; it occurs frequently in women and less often in men)
Symptoms: Increased frequency of urination, often in small quantities; sudden, compelling urge to urinate; a burning sensation when urinating; blood in urine; pain in the lower part of the abdomen; feeling sick.
Treatment: Drinking large quantities of fluids, particularly cranberry juice because it provides acidity; antibiotics, if necessary.
Outlook: No serious damage if treated quickly.

Prostatitis
(Inflammation of the prostate gland in men, often caused by a bacterial infection that has spread from the bladder)
Symptoms: Frequent urination; sudden, compelling urge to urinate; pain when urinating; a frequent, dull pain in the lower part of the abdomen and deep in the pelvis, sometimes accompanied by an urge to move your bowels; the pain often intensifies during urination and sexual intercourse.
Treatment: Antibiotics.
Outlook: May be slow to clear and can recur.

Infants

Urinary tract infections in infants are often associated with abnormalities of the urinary tract that are present at birth. Such disorders increase the possibility of urine flowing backward up the ureter when the bladder is full or during urination. The urine carries bacteria to the kidneys, causing inflammation that can scar the kidneys and lead to kidney failure later in life. Consult your doctor if your child shows symptoms such as nausea or vomiting, frequent urination, or abdominal pain with episodes of crying. Any congenital abnormality may require surgical correction.

Women

Women who are sexually active and use a diaphragm, contraceptive sponge, intrauterine device (IUD), or cervical cap are more susceptible to urinary tract infections. Urinary problems are common in pregnant women, partly because an increase in hormone levels relaxes the muscles in the ureter and bladder. In addition, the enlarged uterus exerts pressure on the bladder, causing an increased need to urinate. Doctors regularly check the urine of pregnant women for bacteria. Untreated urinary tract infections can cause premature labor and can lead to serious complications such as acute pyelonephritis (see page 127), an inflammation of the kidneys.

In older women, falling hormone levels contribute to weakening of the pelvic muscles and slipping (prolapse) of the uterus and urethra. These problems can contribute to urinary tract infections.

WARNING

Infections of the lower part of the urinary tract are fairly common and can often be cured easily. But if these infections are not treated early, or if they do not respond to treatment, they can spread upward to the kidneys, with potentially serious consequences. You should consult your doctor immediately if you or a family member has any symptoms that indicate a urinary tract infection (see page 127).

DIAGNOSING A URINARY TRACT INFECTION

If your doctor suspects that you have a urinary tract infection, he or she will ask you to provide a midstream sample of urine (see below) and may prescribe antibiotics. The specimen will be examined under a microscope for bacteria and the white blood cells that help form pus. A drop of urine then will be placed on a gel containing nutrients that will promote the growth of any disease-causing bacteria. Within a day or two, laboratory staff can identify the bacterium and calculate the number present. Paper disks impregnated with different antibiotics are put onto the gel to determine which drugs kill the bacteria. If necessary, your doctor can then adjust your prescription.

HOW TO TAKE A MIDSTREAM URINE SAMPLE

The doctor will give you a sterile container in which to put your sample.

1 Clean your genital area with a sterile wipe or a clean cloth and soap and water.

2 Pass a small amount of urine into the toilet to clear the bacteria from the opening of the urethra and the external genitals. Then urinate into the sterile container to collect a small sample.

3 You may be asked to label the container with your name. Your sample will be sent to the microbiology laboratory for analysis.

Men

Urinary tract infections are unusual in men until later in life, usually after the age of 50, when the prostate gland enlarges and interferes with emptying of the bladder. When urine stays in the bladder longer than normal, bacteria have an opportunity to multiply and cause infections. Most urinary tract infections in men have an identifiable cause, such as a stone that blocks the flow of urine in the ureter or an enlarged prostate gland.

Bladder inflammation
Viewed through a cystoscope, these two images show a normal bladder lining and an inflamed bladder lining.

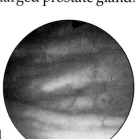

Normal

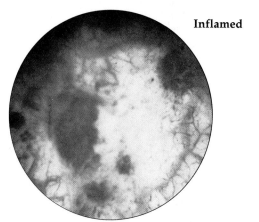

Inflamed

TESTS

In all cases of suspected urinary tract infection, the first step is to test a sample of urine (see page 128). More testing is usually required for men, for women with recurrent infections, and for women whose infections occur above the bladder in the ureter or kidney.

Images of the kidneys may be obtained to determine whether a structural abnormality or blockage is restricting the flow of urine. The doctor may examine the inside of the bladder through a thin viewing tube (called a cystoscope) that is passed up through the urethra. In men, the doctor may perform a rectal examination to determine whether the prostate is infected; women may have a pelvic examination. Blood tests are sometimes used to help evaluate kidney function and screen for diabetes.

TREATMENT

Depending on the infection, an antibiotic may be prescribed as a single dose or for 3 or 7 days. If you have repeated urinary tract infections that appear to be associated with sexual activity, your doctor may recommend that you take an antibiotic immediately after intercourse. Long-term low doses of antibiotics may help prevent recurrent infections.

ANTIBIOTICS

Use these guidelines when you take antibiotics:

◆ Follow the instructions exactly. Do not stop taking the medicine even when your symptoms improve. To eradicate the infection, you must take the entire amount prescribed.

◆ Monitor your symptoms. If they do not improve within 24 hours, you may need to take a different antibiotic to fight the particular bacterium that is causing your infection.

SELF-HELP FOR PREVENTING INFECTION

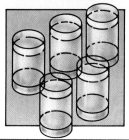

After urinating or having a bowel movement, women should always wipe from front to back to avoid spreading disease-causing organisms from the anus to the bladder.

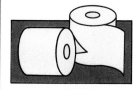

Don't use strong soaps, deodorants, or antiseptic preparations. They can damage the delicate mucous membrane around the opening of the urethra and disrupt your body's natural defenses.

A regular flow of urine prevents bacteria from becoming established in the urinary tract. Keep your bladder empty by making sure that you urinate whenever you have the urge. Do not put off urinating; try to urinate at least every 2 to 4 hours during the day.

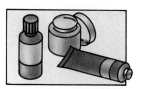

Drink at least 8 to 10 glasses of fluids (preferably water) every day. If you have an infection, drink extra fluids when you awaken during the night. Often people drink less water when they have a urinary tract infection to avoid the discomfort of urinating, but large quantities of fluids help cleanse the urinary tract and reduce the burning sensation.

SEXUALLY TRANSMITTED DISEASES

SEXUALLY TRANSMITTED DISEASES (STDs) have been a common, worldwide problem throughout history. But society's negative attitude toward these infections and reluctance to discuss sexual practices openly have hampered research and the development of improved methods of diagnosis and treatment.

Sexually transmitted diseases are infections that are acquired by exposure to infected body fluids during sexual activities such as vaginal, anal, or, in some cases, oral sex. STDs are increasing at an alarming rate throughout the world.

Who gets STDs?
Any of us can acquire an STD. The incidence of these diseases is higher in some portions of the population, such as .people living in large cities, illicit drug users, prostitutes, people under 25, and people in lower socioeconomic groups.

STOPPING THE SPREAD OF INFECTION

Sexual partners of a person with an STD must be notified so they can receive treatment and avoid spreading the disease. With a disease such as gonorrhea, in which symptoms develop soon after exposure, it is relatively simple to trace partners. But with many STDs, such as AIDS (acquired immune deficiency syndrome), symptoms may not develop for months or even years, making the tracing of partners extremely difficult.

INCIDENCE OF STDS

The incidence of STDs in developed countries declined steadily after World War II, but the development of the contraceptive pill and more open attitudes toward sex in the 1960s and 1970s reversed the trend. In the mid-1980s, the incidence of some STDs declined briefly after the emergence of AIDS, probably because of education and the encouragement of safe sex practices.

Incidence of AIDS in the US
Shown here is the increase in the number of AIDS cases since 1984, as well as a breakdown of the ways in which the disease was acquired.

KEY
☐ Homosexual/bisexual contact
☐ Intravenous drug use
☐ Heterosexual contact
■ Other

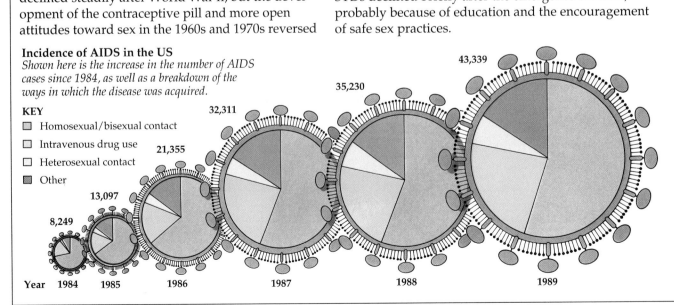

8,249   13,097   21,355   32,311   35,230   43,339

Year   1984   1985   1986   1987   1988   1989

COMMON STDs

The most common sexually transmitted diseases are described on the following pages. Early diagnosis and treatment of these infections are essential because they can have serious long-term or permanent and sometimes even fatal consequences. Gonorrhea can cause infertility in both sexes, chlamydia can cause infertility or abnormal pregnancy in women, and syphilis can lead to severe, permanent physical and mental damage.

Genital herpes

Painful blisters on the genitals may develop within a few days or a few months of exposure to the herpes simplex virus. The blisters clear up quickly, but may recur. Recurrences gradually decrease in severity and frequency.

Genital herpes infections are diagnosed by a physical examination and laboratory analysis of samples taken from blisters. The virus can be treated with the antiviral drug acyclovir. To avoid spreading the infection, a person who has herpes sores should abstain from sex.

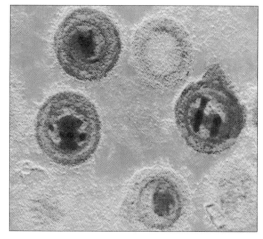

Herpes simplex virus
Genital herpes is caused by the herpes simplex virus (shown in the color-enhanced photograph above, magnified 24,000 times). When the virus infects the mouth area, it causes cold sores. During oral sex, the virus can be spread to the genital area.

Symptoms of genital herpes
Small blisters develop and then break, forming painful ulcers (shown at right). The first infection may be severe, with widespread ulceration in the genital area and symptoms including fever, sore throat, and a headache.

Genital ulcers

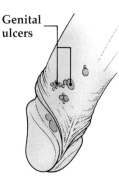

STD CLINICS
Most cities have clinics that specialize in treating STDs. Anyone who suspects he or she has an STD should be tested. Counselors are usually available to help with notification of sexual partners and to discuss the person's concerns about treatment and the long-term consequences of an infection. People undergoing testing for the human immunodeficiency virus (HIV), which causes AIDS, can get help and advice from STD clinics.

Incidence of syphilis and gonorrhea in the US
The bar chart at right shows the incidence of gonorrhea and the combined incidence of primary- and secondary-stage syphilis in the US between 1980 and 1989. The numbers given for each year represent the incidence per 100,000 people.

KEY

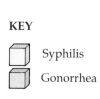

Syphilis

Gonorrhea

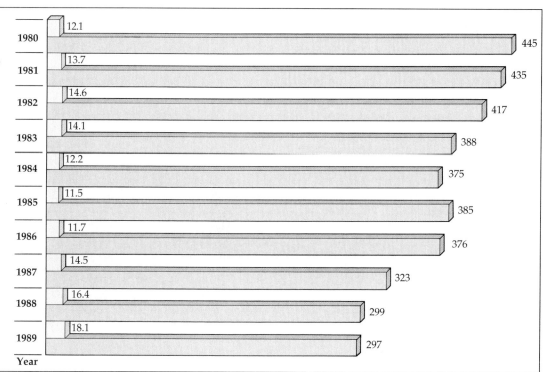

Year	Syphilis	Gonorrhea
1980	12.1	445
1981	13.7	435
1982	14.6	417
1983	14.1	388
1984	12.2	375
1985	11.5	385
1986	11.7	376
1987	14.5	323
1988	16.4	299
1989	18.1	297

Genital warts

Genital warts, caused by the human papillomavirus, are increasingly common in the US. After exposure, months or years may pass before warts develop. Treatment includes applying substances that destroy the warts, freezing or burning them, or removing them surgically. Injecting interferon, an antiviral agent, directly into the skin around the warts may also be effective. Because cervical cancer is more common in women who have had genital warts, they should have a Pap smear at least once a year. Sexual partners should be informed.

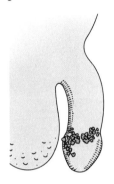

Sites of genital warts
In men, warts occur on the penis (see left) and around the anus. In women, they occur in the vaginal area and around the anus, as well as on the cervix (the neck of the uterus).

SAFE SEX

Following these guidelines can significantly reduce your risk of acquiring an STD:

◆ Have only one sexual partner who has sex only with you.

◆ Use a condom for all penetrating sexual activity.

◆ Avoid sex that may damage a condom or tear the delicate tissue lining the vagina and anus.

◆ Use spermicidal jellies with nonoxynol 9; it may have an antiviral effect.

◆ Use a latex condom during oral sex.

◆ Use water-based lubricants only; oil-based lubricants can damage condoms.

◆ Abstain from sex if you or your partner has symptoms of an STD or is being treated for one.

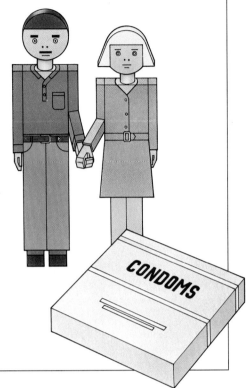

Gonorrhea

In the US, 733,151 cases of gonorrhea were reported in 1989. The symptoms in women are described at right. In men, infection causes a discharge from the penis and pain during urination; rectal infection causes pain and a discharge. Untreated gonorrhea can cause infertility and severe arthritis in both sexes. Anyone who has symptoms, or who has had sexual contact with an infected person, should see a doctor immediately.

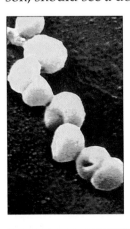

What causes gonorrhea?
Gonorrhea is caused by the bacterium Neisseria gonorrhoeae, *shown in the color-enhanced photograph at left, magnified 13,000 times. The organisms infect the urethra (the tube from the bladder) and rectum in men, and the cervix, uterus, fallopian tubes, urethra, and rectum in women.*

Symptoms of gonorrhea in women
Many women with gonorrhea have no symptoms until complications, such as infections in the uterus and fallopian tubes, develop. Some women have abdominal pain or a vaginal discharge and experience pain during sexual intercourse or a burning sensation when urinating.

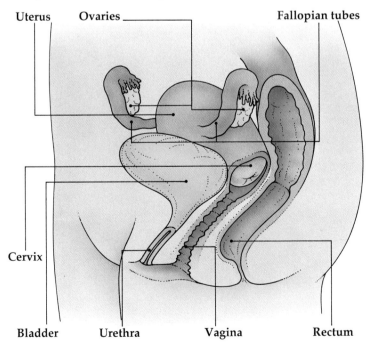

Uterus Ovaries Fallopian tubes

Cervix

Bladder Urethra Vagina Rectum

CASE HISTORY
PAINFUL URINATION

ONE MORNING, **Jeff felt a burning, stinging pain while urinating. He had the same pain repeatedly for the next 2 days. Jeff then noticed a drop of yellow pus at the tip of his penis and stains on his underwear. Alarmed, he immediately went to the health clinic at his college.**

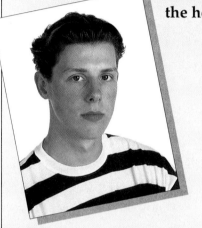

PERSONAL DETAILS
Name Jeff Kline
Age 21
Occupation College student
Family Jeff has two older sisters and a younger one. They are all healthy. Both his parents are well.

MEDICAL BACKGROUND
Jeff is healthy. He has no history of major illnesses.

THE CONSULTATION
After Jeff tells him about his symptoms, the doctor asks about his recent sexual activity. Jeff tells the doctor that in the last 12 days he has had sex with three women and admits that he did not use a condom during any of the encounters. The doctor examines him, takes a sample of the discharge from his penis, and sends it to the laboratory for analysis. The doctor explains that the discharge is probably caused by a sexually transmitted disease.

THE DIAGNOSIS
Microscopic examination of the sample reveals the presence of the organism that causes GONORRHEA. Any of the women that Jeff had sex with could have been the source of his infection. The doctor explains that one out of two women with gonorrhea has no symptoms, so the in-

fected woman could very well be unaware of it. In addition, Jeff may, in turn, have infected the other women he had sex with. The doctor tells Jeff he should inform his sexual partners about the possibility of infection. The doctor schedules Jeff to

Taking precautions
The doctor discusses with Jeff the importance of using condoms during sexual activity to protect himself and his partners from STDs.

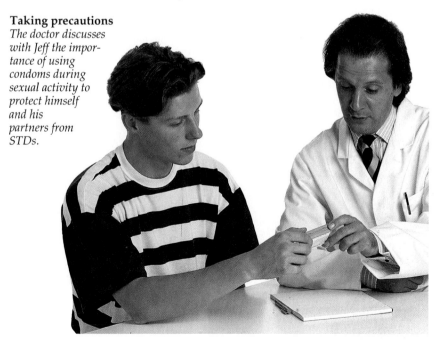

have a blood test for syphilis in case he may have been infected with that STD as well. The doctor also recommends that Jeff be tested for HIV (the virus that causes AIDS) in 3, 6, and 12 months. The test for syphilis is negative.

THE TREATMENT
Jeff is given a single dose of the antibiotic ceftriaxone by injection. He also takes another antibiotic (tetracycline) to treat a possible chlamydia infection (see page 134). Chlamydia infections occur along with half of all cases of gonorrhea.

THE OUTCOME
Jeff's symptoms disappear after a day or two. But the doctor warns Jeff that, especially if he continues to have more than one sexual partner, he must use condoms and follow other safe sex practices during sexual activities to diminish his risk of acquiring and spreading STDs, including AIDS.

Nongonococcal urethritis

Nongonococcal urethritis (inflammation of the urethra) is the name given to urethritis caused by organisms other than those that cause gonorrhea. Most cases of nongonococcal urethritis originate from the same bacterium that causes chlamydia, an STD that affects more than 4 million Americans each year. The symptoms of nongonococcal urethritis, if any, occur slowly and worsen over several days. The infection may produce a discharge of mucus from the urethra and pain when urinating, but, because the initial symptoms are sometimes mild, many people delay seeking medical treatment. However, if the infection spreads in a woman, it can cause pelvic inflammatory disease (infection of the uterus, fallopian tubes, or ovaries) – the most frequent cause of preventable infertility in American women.

In men, nongonococcal urethritis can affect the prostate gland and the epididymis (the small tube that stores sperm

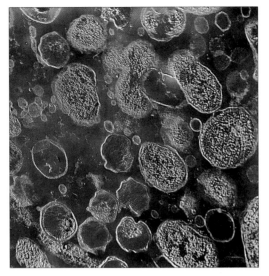

The most common source
The bacterium Chlamydia trachomatis *(the red spheres in the color-enhanced photograph at left, magnified 32,000 times) causes about 30 to 50 percent of cases of nongonococcal urethritis.*

produced in the testicle). It is not known whether nongonococcal urethritis is a cause of infertility in men.

A person with nongonococcal urethritis is treated with an antibiotic such as tetracycline. Sexual partners of infected people should be treated at the same time. During this time, infected people should abstain from sex.

CRAB LICE

Crab lice, or pubic lice, are insects that live in pubic hair and, occasionally, in other areas of the body where hair grows, such as the eyelashes and eyebrows. Crab lice are transmitted by close, usually sexual, contact. The parasites are difficult to remove by scratching or washing because they can lock onto a shaft of hair with their "claws." Crab lice are not dangerous, but they are annoying because they bite the skin to suck blood, which causes itching and irritation. Medication is available to eliminate these parasites.

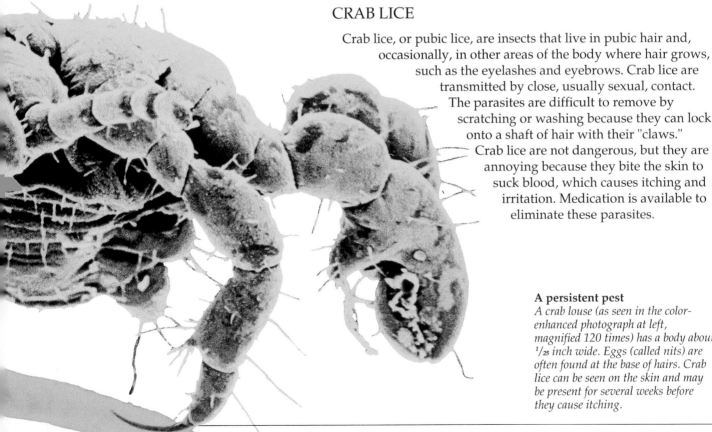

A persistent pest
A crab louse (as seen in the color-enhanced photograph at left, magnified 120 times) has a body about 1/25 inch wide. Eggs (called nits) are often found at the base of hairs. Crab lice can be seen on the skin and may be present for several weeks before they cause itching.

Syphilis

Syphilis was once a widespread illness, feared because of the paralysis and insanity that could result from it. Today, because of effective screening and treatment, it is much less common. Nevertheless, syphilis remains a serious infection, with 44,540 cases of primary and secondary syphilis reported in the US in 1989. If not treated, the disease-causing bacteria can remain in the body indefinitely. The disease has three recognized stages (see below): primary, secondary, and tertiary (or late-stage) syphilis. A person with syphilis is infectious during all stages of the disease. Primary and early secondary syphilis can be cured with penicillin but the effects of late-stage syphilis, including aortic aneurysms (weakened blood vessels) and brain impairment, cannot be reversed. However, treatment can prevent further damage.

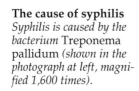

The cause of syphilis
Syphilis is caused by the bacterium Treponema pallidum *(shown in the photograph at left, magnified 1,600 times).*

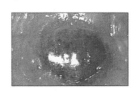

Primary syphilis
Between 9 and 90 days after infection, a painless ulcer develops on the genitals (shown left on the penis) or around the mouth or anus. Without treatment, the ulcer disappears after 6 to 10 weeks.

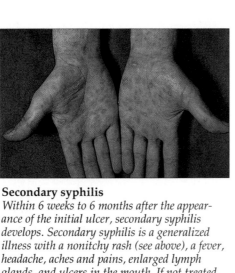

Secondary syphilis
Within 6 weeks to 6 months after the appearance of the initial ulcer, secondary syphilis develops. Secondary syphilis is a generalized illness with a nonitchy rash (see above), a fever, headache, aches and pains, enlarged lymph glands, and ulcers in the mouth. If not treated, the symptoms of secondary syphilis gradually subside and the person moves into a symptomless stage of the disease.

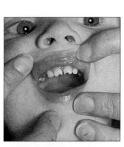

Congenital syphilis
A pregnant woman with untreated syphilis can pass the infection to the fetus via the placenta. Notched teeth (above) are a characteristic of untreated congenital (present at birth) syphilis, which is life-threatening. Congenital syphilis is rare in the US because most pregnant women are screened for the infection and effectively treated.

Tertiary syphilis
If syphilis remains untreated, complications may develop years later. Potential complications include ulceration of the skin and internal organs and damage to bones, the cardiovascular system, spinal cord, and brain (leading to dementia).

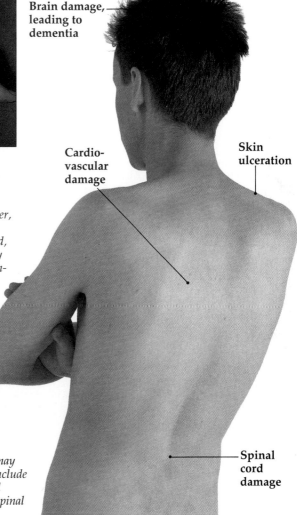

Brain damage, leading to dementia

Cardio-vascular damage

Skin ulceration

Bone damage

Spinal cord damage

HIV INFECTION AND AIDS

AIDS (acquired immune deficiency syndrome), a disease in which the immune system breaks down, was first recognized in 1981. Three years later, a previously unknown virus was identified as the infecting organism. The virus is called HIV (human immunodeficiency virus). There is currently no treatment to inactivate the virus or to cure AIDS. However, by treating HIV-related health problems and using antiviral drugs such as zidovudine (AZT), it is possible to delay the onset of AIDS and prolong survival. The chances of doing so are improved by early detection of the virus. Regularly measuring the level of special white blood cells (called helper T cells) in an infected person's blood gives an indication of the state of his or her immune system. Helper T cells play a key role in orchestrating the body's immune response. If the level of a person's helper T cells is low, he or she is treated to prevent AIDS-related infections, such as pneumocystis carinii pneumonia, a major cause of death in people with AIDS.

COURSE OF HIV INFECTION

HIV invades and replicates inside certain cells of the immune system, gradually weakening its ability to fight infections and cancers. Although it is not known whether all HIV-infected people will develop AIDS, research suggests that most will go through the stages described here. Reported cases of AIDS have so far been consistently fatal.

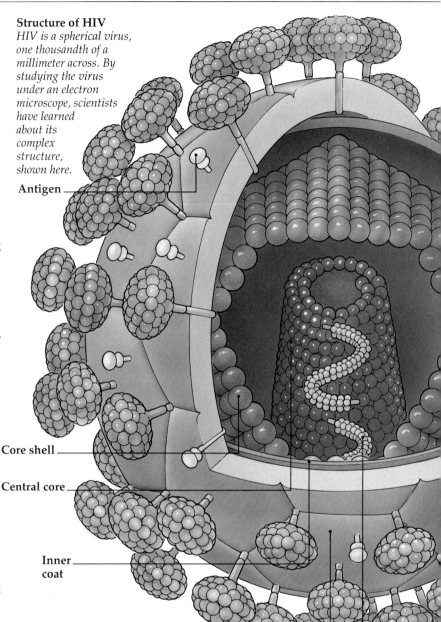

Structure of HIV
HIV is a spherical virus, one thousandth of a millimeter across. By studying the virus under an electron microscope, scientists have learned about its complex structure, shown here.

Antigen

Core shell

Central core

Inner coat

Outer envelope

Genetic material

An infected helper T cell
HIV's main target is the helper T cell, which regulates the function of other immune cells (see page 65). In this color-enhanced photograph (magnified 16,000 times), small particles of HIV (green) are visible on the surface of a helper T cell (white).

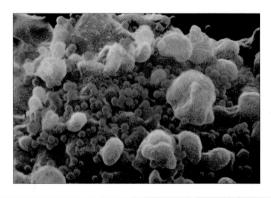

Stage 1: Acute infection
Shortly after HIV infection, one out of four people experiences an illness resembling infectious mononucleosis while the virus replicates inside the body. After a few weeks, the symptoms disappear.

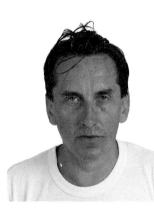

Surface proteins

HOW IS HIV TRANSMITTED?

HIV **can** be transmitted or acquired by:

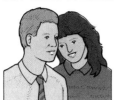 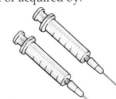 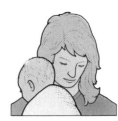

◆ **Sexual contact**
HIV can be transmitted during anal or vaginal intercourse and, possibly, during oral sex. A person with other STDs, particularly genital ulcers, increases his or her risk of infection.

◆ **Infected blood**
Sharing needles to inject intravenous drugs can lead to exposure to blood containing the virus. A small number of health-care workers have been infected through accidental pricks with contaminated needles.

◆ **Mother to baby**
An HIV-infected woman may transmit the virus to her baby during pregnancy or childbirth or sometimes during breast-feeding. One in three babies born to HIV-infected women is infected.

HIV **cannot** be acquired by:

◆ **Nonsexual social contact** Activities such as sharing cups, shaking hands, and kissing cannot transmit the virus.
◆ **Insect bites** Insects do not carry the virus.
◆ **Donating blood** A new sterile needle is used for each donor.

HOW TO AVOID HIV INFECTION

◆ Do not have intercourse with HIV-infected people or people at high risk, such as intravenous drug abusers or people with multiple sex partners.

◆ Practice safe sex (see page 132).

◆ Do not use unsterile needles, whether to inject illegal intravenous drugs or while undergoing tattooing or ear piercing.

◆ Wear protective equipment if your job brings you into contact with blood or blood products.

◆ Bank your own blood before having elective surgery.

Stage 3: Swelling lymph glands
Chronic swelling of lymph glands in the neck, armpits, and other places in the body is often the first sign of HIV infection. Periods of swelling may occur for up to 10 years or more before the development of a full-blown case of AIDS.

Stage 4: Advanced symptoms
Further immune deficiency may lead to:
◆ AIDS-related complex (ARC) – development of symptoms such as weight loss and fatigue and some persistent or recurrent infections that are not considered to indicate a full-blown case of AIDS.
◆ AIDS – identified by specific cancers or opportunistic infections (see page 23) such as yeast infections and pneumocystis pneumonia (a type of pneumonia that causes death in many people with AIDS).
◆ Signs of damage to the nervous system (such as memory loss and dementia).

Persistent or recurrent infections
Recurrent infections of the skin or mucous membranes, such as the yeast infection candidiasis of the mouth (shown below), the vagina, or the esophagus, often accompany HIV infection.

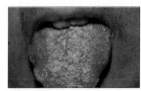

Stage 2: Asymptomatic phase
Once the virus has been established, it may replicate slowly, producing no apparent symptoms for between 2 and 10 years or longer.

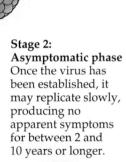

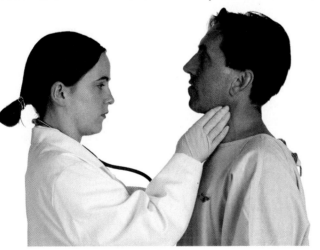

Kaposi's sarcoma
The purple sore shown below is characteristic of Kaposi's sarcoma, a previously rare form of cancer that is the cancer most commonly associated with AIDS.

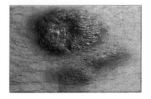

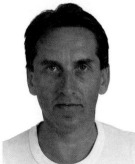

ASK YOUR DOCTOR
STDs

Q **My doctor told me I have nongonococcal urethritis and recommended that my girlfriend have a checkup. She has no symptoms, so is this really necessary?**

A Yes. She should go to her doctor immediately. Initially, nongonococcal urethritis rarely causes symptoms in women. However, the infection can lead to serious complications such as infertility if it is not treated.

Q **I have sores on my penis that are very painful and look like chickenpox. What can they be?**

A Genital herpes is the most likely cause of your rash. After examining you, your doctor may take a sample from a sore for testing. A blood test for syphilis will also be performed. Your doctor may prescribe the antiviral drug acyclovir to heal the sores and relieve your symptoms. You should abstain from sex when you have herpes sores on your penis.

Q **I am gay and have had the same partner for years. Last weekend I had sex with someone else. Should I have an HIV test (for AIDS) right away?**

A A blood test for the virus probably would not show up positive now because it usually takes from 6 weeks to 3 months for the body to produce antibodies to HIV. Have the test in about 5 weeks and again in 3 months, 6 months, and 12 months. Meanwhile, you should abstain from sex or practice safe sex to protect your partner. A person can spread HIV immediately after being infected and before testing postive.

TEENAGERS AND STDs

By age 18, two out of three boys and one out of two girls have had sexual intercourse. Each year, an estimated 3 million American teenagers contract STDs. Many cases go untreated because teens don't know where to go or how to pay for treatment. They are too embarrassed to ask for help and don't want their parents to know. Education should focus on abstinence and/or protection against STDs.

SEXUALLY TRANSMITTED VIRAL HEPATITIS

Hepatitis viruses B and C may be transmitted by sexual intercourse. Although a vaccine for hepatitis B has been available since 1981, the incidence of the disease has increased in the US during the last decade. People in high-risk groups – including male homosexuals, intravenous drug users, prostitutes, and health care workers who come into contact with blood – should get a vaccination. There are no vaccines available for other hepatitis viruses. Hepatitis infections can cause severe complications and occasionally progress to cirrhosis or liver cancer (see page 117). Some people remain highly infectious carriers of the hepatitis B virus for many years.

TRICHOMONIASIS

Trichomoniasis is a common STD that occurs in both men and women, sometimes along with other sexually transmitted diseases. The infection usually does not cause serious problems, but it can be irritating. Women with trichomoniasis may have a watery, greenish, offensive-smelling discharge, and irritation and soreness around the vulva (the external part of the female genitals). They may also have pain during urination and sexual intercourse. Men often have no symptoms, or they may have a discharge from the penis and discomfort while urinating. Trichomoniasis is treated with the antibiotic metronidazole, usually taken for 1 week. You should not drink alcohol while taking this medication. It is important that both partners be treated at the same time to avoid reinfection.

What causes trichomoniasis?
The protozoal parasite Trichomonas vaginalis *(shown in the color-enhanced photograph at right, magnified 7,000 times) causes trichomoniasis. The infection is diagnosed by identification of the organism under a microscope.*

CASE HISTORY
UNUSUAL GROWTHS

AFTER TAKING A SHOWER one morning, Teresa was shocked to find fleshy warts around her vagina. She thought at first that the growths would go away by themselves, but instead they continued to increase in number and size over the next few weeks. Teresa made an appointment to see her doctor right away.

PERSONAL DETAILS
Name Teresa Belmont
Age 41
Occupation Journalist
Family Both of Teresa's parents are dead. She has a younger brother, who is healthy.

MEDICAL BACKGROUND
Teresa's general health is good. She had appendicitis as an adolescent, but no other major illnesses.

THE CONSULTATION
The doctor listens while Teresa describes her problem and then he examines her. He finds that Teresa's labia (the folds of skin around the vagina) and vagina are covered with flat, fleshy, cauliflowerlike growths that extend to the area around her anus. When questioned, Teresa says that the growths have been itching and that she has had some pain during urination.

After the operation
The gynecologist explains to Teresa that if any warts start to regrow, he will treat them with a powerful liquid medication. He recommends that she return for treatment whenever new warts appear.

THE DIAGNOSIS
The doctor tells Teresa that she has GENITAL WARTS, which are usually acquired from an infected person during sexual intercourse. Teresa explains that she has had only one partner in 5 years and she is no longer seeing him because she found out he was having sex with other women. The doctor says that he must be the source of the infection. He refers Teresa to a gynecologist.

THE GYNECOLOGIST'S CONSULTATION
The gynecologist explains that the human papillomavirus makes some body cells grow abnormally, producing warts. The warts themselves are not cancerous, but women who have had genital warts are more likely to develop cancer of the cervix. The gynecologist explains to Teresa that, although the warts can be removed, the virus may not be completely eliminated.

THE TREATMENT
Teresa's warts are removed surgically by burning (diathermy) while she is under general anesthesia. The gynecologist asks Teresa to return in 3 weeks, when she will no longer be sore from the operation. He tells her he will then apply medication to any warts that start to regrow.

THE OUTCOME
After several months, the warts are gone. However, the gynecologist cannot guarantee that Teresa is no longer infectious or that the warts will not recur. Teresa decides to use condoms during sex. Her gynecologist recommends that she have an annual Pap smear from now on to screen for cervical cancer.

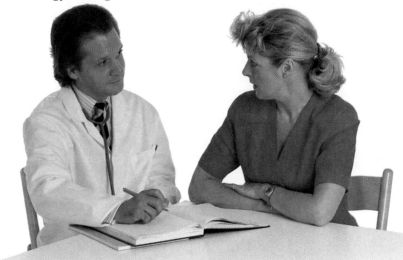

139

GLOSSARY OF INFECTIOUS DISEASES

Many major infectious diseases covered in this volume are not listed in the glossary. See the index on pages 142 to 144.

A

Anthrax
A rare infectious disease of farm animals caused by a bacterium. Anthrax occasionally spreads to people, usually causing a skin infection. The spores of the bacteria can lie dormant in the soil for many years.

Aspergillosis
A lung infection caused by a fungus found in decaying plants and old buildings. Aspergillosis is spread by airborne spores. The infection is rare in healthy people but more common and potentially fatal in a person with an impaired immune system, such as someone who is undergoing chemotherapy for cancer.

B

Babesiosis
A rare infectious disease caused by a protozoal parasite of rodents and horses. The disease is transmitted to humans by tick bites. The symptoms, which include fever and chills, closely resemble those of malaria. No specific treatment is available.

Blastomycosis
A rare lung infection caused by a fungus found in rotting wood and soil. Blastomycosis may cause acute or chronic pneumonia or a long-term illness that affects the lungs, skin, and bones.

Botulism
A rare but serious type of food poisoning acquired by eating improperly preserved or canned food that is contaminated with a powerful toxin produced by a type of bacterium.

Brucellosis
A now uncommon bacterial infection acquired from farm animals or their milk. The bacteria are inhaled or ingested, or enter the bloodstream through breaks in the skin. Unpasteurized dairy products are another source of infection.

C-D

Chagas' disease
An infectious disease found in South and Central America that is spread by insects called cone-nose or assassin bugs. The disease-causing parasites travel in the bloodstream and can affect the esophagus, heart, intestines, and central nervous system.

Chancroid
A sexually transmitted disease that is common in the tropics. It is caused by a bacterium that produces painful ulcers on the genitals and enlarged lymph nodes in the groin. The infection can be treated with antibiotics.

Coccidioidomycosis
A lung infection (also called San Joaquin Valley fever) acquired by inhaling airborne fungal spores. Symptoms occur in only 40 percent of infected people and range from a mild illness to severe pneumonia. If the disease does not subside on its own, it can be treated with antifungal drugs.

Cryptococcosis
A rare infection acquired by inhaling a fungus. Cryptococcosis is more common in people whose immune systems are weakened, such as people with AIDS. The infection can cause meningitis (inflammation of the membranes that cover the brain and spinal cord), pneumonia, and growths on the skin.

Cysticercosis
A rare infection that occurs when pork tapeworm larvae invade tissues in the body, after a person accidentally swallows the eggs of an adult pork tapeworm. Infection causes cysts to develop in body tissues.

Dengue
A tropical disease caused by a virus carried by mosquitoes. The illness is characterized by a sudden onset of chills, fever, and severe headaches that last for a few days. A brief remission is followed by fever, pains, and a red rash all over the body that may resemble measles.

H

Histoplasmosis
An infection acquired by inhaling the spores of a fungus found in soil contaminated with bird or bat droppings. In people with weakened immune systems, it can be chronic with fever, weight loss, mouth ulcers, swollen lymph glands, and anemia.

Hydatid disease
A rare infestation caused by the larval stage of a type of tapeworm usually found in dogs. The larvae settle in the lungs, liver, brain, and other organs, where they form cysts. In the brain, the cysts may cause seizures or paralysis.

L

Lassa fever
A dangerous viral infection, confined mainly to West Africa and believed to be spread to humans from rats, although person-to-person spread has also been reported. The symptoms include chills, fever, headache, pains, and severe vomiting and diarrhea. About one third of all cases are fatal.

Legionnaires' disease
A life-threatening form of pneumonia that is caused by a bacterium that sometimes contaminates water and air-conditioning systems. The initial symptoms include headache, muscular and abdominal pain, diarrhea, and a dry cough, followed by pneumonia, fever, and chills.

Leprosy
A chronic infectious disease caused by a bacterium similar to the one that causes tuberculosis. Leprosy primarily affects the nerves in the arms and legs and face, leading to loss of sensation and disfigurement. The organism may be inhaled or enter the body through the skin. Leprosy is acquired only after many years of exposure to an infected person.

Leptospirosis
A rare disease caused by a spiral-shaped bacterium carried by rats and excreted in their urine. Leptospirosis causes an acute illness with fever, chills, headache, muscle aches, and skin rash. The kidneys may be affected severely; liver damage along with jaundice is common.

Listeriosis
A bacterial infection common in livestock that also occurs in humans. The disease is caused by a bacterium that is transmitted in undercooked meat, soft cheeses, or other foods. Listeriosis can be life-threatening in infants and the elderly. If a pregnant woman is infected, her baby may be stillborn.

Lyme disease
An uncommon infectious disease caused by a bacterium that is transmitted by tick bites. The disease – first recognized in Old Lyme, Connecticut, in 1975 – causes a rash, shortness of breath, and inflammation and swelling of the joints.

O-P

Osteomyelitis
An infection of the bones and bone marrow, usually caused by bacteria that have spread through the bloodstream or from an infection in the skin overlying the bone. The bacteria may enter the bloodstream through a cut in the skin or an infection elsewhere in the body. The blood-borne form of the disease is most common in children and often affects the long bones of the arms and legs.

Pertussis
An infectious bacterial disease (also known as whooping cough) that affects young children and infants. The disease is characterized by paroxysms of coughing that end with a "whoop" as breath is inhaled. Since the development of the pertussis vaccine, the number of deaths from pertussis has fallen.

Poliomyelitis
A now rare infectious disease caused by a virus. Poliomyelitis involves the central nervous system and usually produces only a mild illness. In serious cases, paralysis and sometimes death result. The disease has now been vir-

tually eliminated in the US and Europe as a result of the introduction of vaccines in the 1950s.

Psittacosis
A rare respiratory illness resembling influenza that is caused by a chlamydia species of bacteria and is spread by parrots, pigeons, poultry, and other birds. The disease is acquired by inhaling dust contaminated with infected bird droppings and is most common in farmers and owners of parrots and cockatiels.

Q-R

Q fever
A rare disease caused by rickettsia bacteria that are carried by farm animals. Q fever may be contracted by inhaling contaminated dust particles or from tick bites. People with Q fever develop a flulike illness that can lead to pneumonia, hepatitis, and endocarditis (inflammation of the lining of the heart).

Rheumatic fever
An inflammatory disease that follows a streptococcal infection. Because of antibiotics, it is no longer common.

Rocky Mountain spotted fever
An infectious disease caused by rickettsia bacteria that is transmitted to people by the bites of ticks that have lived on infected rabbits or other small mammals. The illness is characterized by small pink spots on the wrists and ankles, which spread over the entire body and darken, enlarge, and bleed. The disease usually subsides within 2 weeks but can be fatal if not treated.

S

Schistosomiasis
A tropical parasitic disease, also known as bilharziasis, caused by flukes called schistosomes.

Schistosomiasis can be acquired from bathing in infested water. Visitors to countries where the disease is endemic should avoid swimming in rivers or lakes. Salt water, however, is safe to swim in. The infestation causes bleeding and the formation of scar tissue inside the bladder, intestines, or other organs, including the liver and lungs.

Sleeping sickness
A serious infection, also called trypanosomiasis, that is caused by a protozoal parasite. Sleeping sickness is common in tropical Africa where it is spread through the bites of tsetse flies. In humans, the parasites multiply and spread via the bloodstream to other organs. Untreated, the disease is fatal.

Sporotrichosis
A chronic skin infection caused by a fungus and most common in gardeners and florists. The fungus enters the skin through a cut and causes ulceration and formation of nodules. The infection is treated with potassium iodide or antifungal drugs.

T-Y

Tetanus
A serious disease of the central nervous system caused by wounds infected with spores of a bacterium. Tetanus is also known as lockjaw, because it causes spasms of the jaw muscles that make opening the mouth difficult. Other symptoms of tetanus include widespread muscle spasms that can be fatal if the respiratory muscles are affected.

Toxic shock syndrome
A rare condition caused by a toxin produced by a staphylococcus bacterium. The condition has been associated with the use of highly absorbent tampons, which have been removed from the market. Some cases have been linked to prolonged use of a contraceptive diaphragm. Toxic shock causes a high fever, vomiting, diarrhea, headache, muscular pain, dizziness, and a rash resembling a sunburn. Complications include lung, liver, and kidney failure, and death.

Trichinosis
An infestation with the larvae of a worm that is acquired by eating undercooked pork. The larvae, which are released inside the digestive tract, can travel to other organs, particularly muscles, where they settle. Heavy infestation produces diarrhea, vomiting, fever, muscle pain, and swelling around the eyelids.

Tularemia
An infectious disease of wild rabbits, squirrels, and muskrats that is occasionally transmitted to humans. The bacteria that cause tularemia can enter the human body through open skin or the bites of ticks and fleas. The illness is characterized by ulceration at the site of infection, and enlarged lymph glands, headache, muscle pain, and fever. Tularemia is fatal in 5 percent of cases. A vaccine is now available for people who are at risk, such as hunters and laboratory workers.

Typhoid fever
A serious disease caused by a bacterium that is transmitted in food or water contaminated with infected feces. The illness, which lasts about 4 weeks, produces symptoms that include a high fever, headache, and abdominal pain, followed by a rash and diarrhea. If not treated, typhoid fever can be fatal.

Typhus
A group of diseases caused by rickettsia bacteria that are spread by insects such as lice and fleas, and by mites. Epidemic typhus is spread from one person to another by body lice. Endemic typhus is a disease of rats that can be spread to humans by fleas. Scrub typhus is transmitted by mites. If not treated, typhus can be fatal.

Yellow fever
A tropical infectious disease caused by a virus carried by a type of mosquito. The disease is characterized by jaundice, a high fever, nausea, and internal bleeding, especially in the stomach, which results in black vomit. Yellow fever can be fatal.

INDEX

Page numbers in *italics* refer to illustrations and captions.

Photograph sources:
Ardea London Ltd **94** (center left)
Baylor College of Medicine, Houston **33** (bottom left)
Biophoto Associates **22** (center top); **42** (bottom right); **78** (top right); **78** (top center); **93** (center); **97** (bottom right); **135** (top left)
Bridgeman Art Library **27** (bottom right)
Bubbles Photo Library **55** (top left)
Centers for Disease Control **26** (center); **30** (bottom right)
The Environmental Picture Library **71** (center right)
Mary Evans Picture Library **27** (top left)
The Image Bank **33** (bottom right); **58** (top right); **68** (bottom); **71** (bottom right); **81**; **98** (bottom right)
E. Lyon, MD, University of Chicago **129**
National Medical Slide Bank, UK **52** (center right); **89** (center left); **101**; **102** (bottom right); **117** (center); **121** (top left); **122** (top left); **122** (bottom left); **122** (bottom center); **124** (top left); **135** (bottom left)
Oxford Scientific Films **26** (center left); **94** (bottom right)
The Photographers' Library **9**; **61**
Pictor International Ltd **15** (center); **90** (bottom right)
R. G. Ramsey, MD, University of Chicago **95** (center right)
Saint Bartholomew's Hospital **15** (top

right); **86** (center); **89** (top center); **103** (top right); **103** (bottom right); **105** (bottom right); **123** (center right); **124** (bottom right); **135** (center)
Saint Mary's Hospital **14** (center); **86** (bottom left); **109** (top right); **121** (bottom right); **122** (center right); **135** (top right)
Science Photo Library **2** (center left); **2** (bottom right); **7**; **10** (top right); **11** (bottom left); **12** (top left); **12** (bottom right); **13** (top left); **13** (center); **14** (top left); **14** (top right); **18** (center left); **20** (center); **21** (bottom right); **22** (top center); **22** (right); **23** (center); **24** (center left); **26** (top right); **28** (bottom right); **35**; **37**; **39** (bottom); **40**; **41**; **42** (center right); **42** (top center); **43**; **49**; **50**; **52** (bottom left); **52** (center); **55** (bottom right); **57** (top right); **58** (center); **58** (bottom left); **59** (center); **62**; **63**; **64**; **65**; **77**; **78** (center); **78** (bottom right); **83**; **86** (top right); **89** (bottom left); **90** (top left); **96** (center right); **97** (top right); **100** (bottom right); **103** (center); **107** (center); **109** (top left); **111**; **116**; **123** (center left); **131**; **132**; **134**; **136** (bottom)
Tony Stone Worldwide **86** (bottom)
James C. Webb **12** (center); **13** (bottom right); **56** (bottom left); **57** (top center); **59** (center); **112** (bottom center); **115** (center); **125** (bottom); **135** (top left)

World Health Organization **29** (top right)
Zefa **94** (top center); **130**

The photograph on page 76 was taken on the premises of The Aviary, London

**Front cover photograph:
Julian Calder/ Tony Stone Worldwide**

Illustrators:
David Ashby
Russell Barnet
Tony Bellue
Karen Cochrane
David Fathers
Tony Graham
Andrew Green
Guy Smith
Lydia Umney
Philip Wilson
John Woodcock

Commissioned photography:
Steve Bartholomew
Susannah Price

Airbrushing:
Janos Marffy
Richard Manning

Index: Sue Bosanko